AN ETHICAL EVALUATION OF FETAL EXPERIMENTATION:
An Interdisciplinary Study

Edited By Donald G. McCarthy and Albert S. Moraczewski, O. P.

A Report of The Task Force on Fetal Experimentation
Pope John XXIII Medical-Moral
Research and Education Center
St. Louis, Missouri

This book is dedicated to the Charter Members of the Pope John XXIII Center, whose support has made this study possible.

We would like to express grateful appreciation to the following for permission to use quoted material:

Confraternity of Christian Doctrine, Inc., for scripture texts used from the New American Bible, copyright © 1970, by the Confraternity of Christian Doctrine, Washington, D.C. All rights reserved. Rev. Msgr. Vincent A. Yzermans for excerpts from his copyrighted book, *Major Addresses of Pope Pius XII,* North Central Publishing Co., St. Paul, Minnesota. America Press, for excerpts from *The Documents of Vatican II,* reprinted with permission of America Press. All rights reserved. Copyright © 1966, by America Press, 106 W. 56 Street, New York, New York 10019. TPS Publications, for material from "Declaration on Abortion," *The Pope Speaks* (Vol 19, No. 3). T & T Clark, Ltd., for excerpts from *Church Dogmatics* by Karl Barth (Vol. III). Harper & Row Publishers, Inc., for quoted material from *The Ethics of Sex* by Helmut Thielicke. Macmillan Publishing Co., Inc., and SCM Press, Ltd., for material quoted from *Ethics* by Dietrich Bonhoeffer, copyright © 1955. The Christian Century Foundation, excerpt from "What Does Theology Say About Abortion?" by J. Robert Nelson, *The Christian Century* (90: 124-8) Jan. 31, 1973. *The Perkins Journal* for material quoted from the article, "The Beginnings of Personhood: Philosophical Considerations," (*27:* 20-27) Fall, 1973. Willard Gaylin, M.D. and Marc Lappé for quoted material from their copyrighted article, "Fetal Politics," *The Atlantic Monthly,* (*235:* 66-71) May, 1975. A. W. Liley, KCMG, for quoted material from "The Foetus As A Personality," Australian & New Zealand Journal of Psychiatry (6: 99-105) 1972.

IMPRIMI POTEST:
Gerard B. Cleator, O.P.
Provincial

IMPRIMATUR:
† John J. Cardinal Carberry
Archbishop of St. Louis
April 27, 1976

The Pope John XXIII Medical-Moral
Research and Education Center
St. Louis, Missouri 63104

Library of Congress Catalog Card Number: 76-21165

Contents

Prologue

About The Pope John Center

The Pope John XXIII Medical-Moral Research and Education Center was founded in 1973 to provide the Church with carefully documented research studies dealing with the long-range ethical implications of modern medicine and their significance in relation to biotechnological advances. The Center seeks to engage highly competent scientists, physicians, theologians, and ethicists for specific projects. Without adopting a narrow sectarian point of view, the Pope John Center strives to view the relevant ethical and theological issues in the light of Catholic teaching.

About This Report

The practice of fetal experimentation has recently become a focus of increasing concern. The recent Supreme Court decision that legalized abortion has apparently led to an unprecedented, and inadequately anticipated situation of increased availability of human fetuses for medical research.

In its consideration of fetal experimentation, the Christian Church faces a unique dilemma: As an advocate of the powerless, the Church strives to protect the human fetus from abuse, while, in its equally important role of promoting human well-being, the Church also recognizes the need for medical research involving the fetus for the improvement of perinatal care. How is this tension to be resolved?

To respond to the question thoughtfully, the Pope John Center sponsored a Task Force on Fetal Experimentation from which emanated this study. It is in light of that tension-question that the present study seeks to analyze the ethical issues involved in fetal experimentation and to discover the valid foundations for a broadly based consensus concerning our need as a human, civilized community to protect the fetus. The study critically reviews the recommendations of the National Commission for the Protection of Human Subjects of Biomedical and Behavioral Research and the current published policy of the federal government as reflected in the Regulations of The Department of Health, Education and Welfare, which regulates the funding of fetal research. It proposes some alternative guidelines more acceptable to Christian thought and, we believe, to the informed general public.

And, finally, because the medieval theory of "mediate animation" (delayed hominization) has recently gained new prominence and seems to be exercising what we believe to be a quite unwarranted influence, we include a detailed discussion of this subject in an appendix. It should be noted that the ethical argument and conclusions of this report are independent of the rejection or acceptance of this theory.

Task Force Members

Benedict Ashley, OP, PhD
Professor of Moral Theology
The Aquinas Institute of Theology
Dubuque, Iowa

Joseph Bracken, SJ, PhD
Associate Professor
Department of Theology
Marquette University
Milwaukee, Wisconsin

Paul Byrne, MD
Director
Newborn Intensive Care Unit
Cardinal Glennon Memorial Hospital For Children
St. Louis, Missouri
&
Associate Clinical Professor
Department of Pediatrics
St. Louis University School of Medicine
St. Louis, Missouri

Fernando de Castro, MD
Associate Professor
Departments of Pediatrics and Community Medicine
St. Louis University School of Medicine
St. Louis, Missouri
&
Director
Ambulatory Services
Cardinal Glennon Memorial Hospital For Children
St. Louis, Missouri

Betty Gaiss, OP
Graduate Assistant
Department of Human Development
College of Human Medicine
Michigan State University
Lansing, Michigan

Donald McCarthy, PhD
Professor of Christian Ethics
Mount St. Mary's Seminary of the West
Norwood, Ohio
&
Visiting Lecturer in Medical Ethics
Institute of Religion
Texas Medical Center
Houston, Texas

Albert Moraczewski, OP, PhD
President
Pope John XXIII Medical-Moral Research and Education Center
St. Louis, Missouri
&
Adjunct Associate Professor of Ethics
St. Louis University School of Medicine
St. Louis, Missouri
&
Visiting Associate Professor of Ethics
Baylor College of Medicine
Houston, Texas

Kevin O'Rourke, OP, JCD
Director
Medical Moral Affairs
The Catholic Hospital Association
St. Louis, Missouri
&
Professor of Moral and Pastoral Theology
The Aquinas Institute of Theology
Dubuque, Iowa

Maurice Zeller, CSSR, PhD (Consultant)
St. Louis University
St. Louis, Missouri
&
Professor of Moral Theology
Mount St. Alphonsus Seminary
Esopus, NY

Acknowledgements

A project such as this one depends on the assistance of numerous people. Grateful thanks are due The Board of Trustees of the Catholic Hospital Association for having established, and initially funded the Pope John XXIII Medical-Moral Research and Education Center. In addition, this entire project was made possible by the constant and active support of The Catholic Hospital Association, whose various staff members, in a number of different ways, have assisted the functioning of the Center and the Task Force; to them all we express our gratitude.

We express our thanks to The Board of Directors of the Pope John Center for their enthusiastic and ever present encouragement of this Study.

Central to this project, of course, is the Task Force which produced this document. As editors of the Study, we wish to state our deep appreciation to each member of the Task Force for his participation in the many meetings and discussions which helped to produce and integrate the work. Each member devoted many days of labor in preparation both for the meetings and for their respective written contributions. Particular recognition is due to Fr. Benedict Ashley, O.P., whose dissertation on delayed hominization in Appendix I constitutes an invaluable addition to this Study. Throughout the text, the source of the brilliant insight, the incisive expression, the felicitous phrasing, remains anonymous, since drafts were circulated several times among the members for comments and corrections. To each and to all we extend our heartfelt thanks, while at the same time we must claim responsibility for errors made subsequent to the submission of the individual manuscripts.

Naturally, this final report itself has gone through several revisions. In particular, we wish to thank those who have carefully read the manuscript at various stages and made significant suggestions. We are very grateful for the supportive comments of members of our Episcopal Advisory Committee who read the entire manuscript in its penultimate form: the Most Reverend George Ahr, (Trenton), the Most Reverend Mark Hurley (Santa Rosa), the Most Reverend Edward D.

Head (Buffalo), and the Most Reverend Maurice Dingman (Des Moines). Special thanks are due John Wakefield, whose astute and scholarly criticisms kept us honest. Excellent suggestions were made by Sister Ann Neale, GNSH, Director, Bishops' Committee for Human Values; Fr. Richard A. McCormick, SJ, Rose F. Kennedy, Professor of Christian Ethics, Center for Bioethics, Georgetown University, and George A. Curran, SJ, Xavier University (Cincinnati). From their special vantage point, two neonatologists on the staff of St. Mary's Hospital Medical Center (Madison, Wisconsin), Angela Skelton, MD, and Elizabeth Purkett, MD, made very insightful remarks. In addition, several individuals read portions of the manuscript and rendered valuable comments. Father Benedict Viviano, OP, Assistant Professor of New Testament, The Aquinas Institute of Theology (Dubuque), and Fr. Eugene Maly, Professor of Biblical Studies, Mount St. Mary's Seminary of the West (Cincinnati) contributed helpful comments on various portions of Chapter IV.

However, in no way do we wish to state or imply that all these individuals agreed with us on every point. Rather, their comments, accepted or rejected, all helped to sharpen our thinking and clarify our expression.

In preparation of the final version of this Study, considerable and valuable editorial input came from Ms. Eleanor L. Schreiner. Her perceptive comments and questions challenged us to express ourselves as clearly and concisely as possible. Under her scrutiny the manuscript emerged more clearly and neatly. To her, our sincere thanks.

We would also like to thank Mr. Ray Mangin for his technical and artistic assistance with the layout, design and cover illustration of this book.

Much gratitude needs to be expressed to those young ladies that patiently typed and retyped the manuscript, often working from difficult-to-read, marked-up sheets of paper: Ms. Deborah Wood, Mrs. Debra Fitzgerald and Miss Vivian Gilbreth. To the last mentioned, thanks are also in order for her meticulous checking of footnotes and references.

To all the above mentioned persons, and to any others, who, because of the frailty of human memory, may have been overlooked, we extend our grateful acknowledgements.

Rev. Donald G. McCarthy
Rev. Albert S. Moraczewski, O.P.
St. Louis, Missouri
February 29, 1976

Introduction

The Public Controversy on Fetal Experimentation

On Friday, August 8, 1975, in the *Federal Register,* new rules and regulations were published which govern the protection of certain human subjects, namely, human fetuses, pregnant women, and the products of human *in vitro* fertilization, to the extent that they are involved in research and related activities supported or conducted by the Department of Health, Education, and Welfare.[1] Thus has ended one phase of an intense public debate involving government policy and the human fetus.

For several years previous to the publication of these regulations, the scientific and public press carried articles strongly affirming the need for fetal experimentation. Other equally emphatic articles declared that such activities were not only unnecessary, but were actually opposed to the public well-being. It is common experience that in such an atmosphere of heated controversy all parties have difficulty reaching a balanced judgment because opposing viewpoints tend to be overstated, leading to partisan polarization. Notwithstanding the difficulties and complexities of the problem, it was clear that some kind of action was necessary at the highest level of government.

Accordingly, on July 12, 1974, the National Research Act (P.L. 93-348) was signed into law. One of its provisions created a National Commission for the Protection of Human Subjects of Biomedical and Behavioral Research and gave it the mandate to conduct studies regarding research on fetuses (and other human subjects) and to make recommendations to the Secretary of the Department of Health, Education, and Welfare (DHEW). Another provision of the National Research Act regarding human fetuses was to declare a moratorium on "research (conducted or supported by DHEW) in the United States or abroad on a living human fetus, before or after the induced abortion of such fetus, unless such research is done for the purpose of assuring the survival of such a fetus."[2]

The National Commission was duly appointed by President Gerald Ford on September 10, 1974. It consisted of eleven members: eight men and three women; by profession there were three physicians, three attorneys, two psychologists, two ethicists and one non-specialist.[3] Whether or not the specific composition of the Commission was representative of the concerned parties might be debated. But, in any event, it was seen as an unprecedented effort on the part of the United States government to confront a complex and controversial ethical question. The meetings were open to the public and all documentation, reports, and verbatim transcripts became part of the published record of the Commission.

On May 21, 1975, the National Commission submitted to the Secretary of DHEW its recommendations regarding fetal research, approximately five months after it was sworn into office on December 3, 1974. During these months, the Commission listened to testimony by a variety of witnesses representing many diverse groups, evaluated a number of lengthy reports containing research for which it contracted, including essays by eight different ethicists and two attorneys, and also reviewed the volumes of mail sent by interested parties. The Commission has now turned its attention to other matters, but there are ramifications of the fetal research issue that need further exploration.

Objective of This Study

In January, 1975, as the National Commission was beginning its work, the Pope John XXIII Medical-Moral Research and Education Center formed a task force to study the issue of fetal experimentation from a perspective different from that of the National Commission and in a manner consistent with its own mandate to study emerging biomedical issues from the point of view of Catholic teaching. Numerous books and articles dealing with the ethical questions attendant to the utilization of human fetuses in medical research were already available in the literature.[4] In addition, the National Conference of Catholic Bishops issued a statement through Monsignor James McHugh, first at the Congressional hearings, and secondly at the public hearings held by the Commission on February 14, 1975, regarding its attitude on the issue.[5] These and many other publications were reviewed by the task force. In addition, relevant teachings of the Holy See were carefully examined for specific statements pertaining to the values which the Church seeks to promote or protect in regard to human life, medical research, and the reciprocal obligations of man in society. Furthermore, the study sought to identify those values of Western culture where, at least, a broad base of consensus was possible.

Research in preparation for this study supported the opinion of an apparent widespread consensus that the human fetus is endowed with a basic human dignity worthy of protection by the adult community. However, such a consensus does not necessarily indicate agreement as to the kind and degree of protection, only that some protection is necessary. Consequently, in view of the fact that there were claims and counterclaims regarding the indispensability of fetal research for societal benefits, it was concluded that a valid ethical analysis would have to proceed within the context of community.

This study, therefore, seeks to explore the issue of the fetus' status in the human community. Consequently, the ethical evaluation of fetal experimentation made here, which can be the basis of an expanding public consensus, is made in terms of those values to which the Catholic Church is committed by its authentic teaching, those which it shares in large measure with all Christian churches and with many other groups dedicated to the service of human rights.

Overview of This Study

In accordance with this aim, the first chapter will discuss fetal experimentation and the ethical challenges it poses. The next three chapters will develop in some detail three converging lines of analysis:

1. *Fetal experimentation and the civic community.* This approaches the issue from the point of view of the human community and the reciprocal relationships existing among the members and between the individual and the group.
2. *Fetal experimentation and the community of persons.* The perspective here is that of a personalist humanism and rests on a philosophical and psychological analysis of personhood.
3. *Fetal experimentation and the Christian community.* This third analysis examines the issues in the light of Biblical sources and the major Christian traditions.

It will be seen that each of these three lines of argumentation, though proceeding from different points of departure, and continuing on different levels of reflection, tend to converge to the consensus mentioned above, namely that the fetus possesses a fundamental human dignity with significant implications for fetal experimentation.

The fifth chapter of this study presents a reflection on the several core ethical issues consequent upon the human dignity of the fetus. The final chapter includes both a detailed analysis of the recommendations formulated by the National Commission for the Protection of Human Subjects of Biomedical and Behavioral Research and a section which reviews the current Regulations published by the Department of Health, Education, and Welfare. Recommendations are proposed as a basis for alternative guidelines, which, it is believed, the Christian community and its pastors could actively promote. Final observations about achieving wider support of such guidelines conclude the chapter. Appendix I analyzes in detail the issue of delayed hominization of the human embryo; Appendix II lists a proposed revision of the National Commission's recommendations in a form which may be more acceptable to those who affirm the personhood of the fetus.

Footnotes

1. *Federal Register,* "Protection of Human Subjects", 40(154):33526 ff., August 8, 1975.
2. *Ibid.,* p. 33531.
3. See *Science* 186:38, October 4, 1974.
4. For example, Ramsey, Paul, *The Ethics of Fetal Research,* New Haven: The Yale University Press, 1975; Etzioni, Amitai, *Genetic Fix,* New York: Macmillan Publishing Co., 1973; Reback, Gary L., "Fetal Experimentation: Moral, Legal and Medical Implications", *Stanford Law Review* 26:1191-1207, May 1974; Walters, LeRoy, "Ethical Issues in Experimentation on the Human Fetus", *Journal of Religious Ethics* 2:33-54, Spring, 1974: Krol, John Cardinal and Berliner, Dr. Robert, "Human Life in the Laboratory", Statements on Fetal Research in the United States, Bishops' Pro-Life Committee, *Origins* 2(44): 698 and 708, April 26, 1973; Hurley, Bishop Mark, "Science and Ethics in a New Age", *Origins* 2(23):365, 367, 377, November 30, 1972.
5. Proceedings of the National Commission for the Protection of Human Subjects of Biomedical and Behavioral Research, (Verbatim transcripts) pp. 201-213, Feb. 14-15, 1975; see also *Origins* 4(9): 138-139, August 15, 1974; see also McHugh, Msgr. James, "Experiments and the Fetus: Why the Opposition?" *Origins* 3(17):268-9, October 18, 1973.

1

Fetal Experimentation and the Challenge of Ethical Concerns

Fetal Experimentation in the Past Decade

Research activity in neonatology and fetology has resulted in many advances in the understanding of fetal development and in the medical care of young patients. Considerable information has been obtained in the past by procedures which most persons would consider to be ethically acceptable, assuming appropriate informed consent. These procedures included: the use of innovative efforts to treat and benefit a particular fetus afflicted with some abnormality that is not amenable to standard medical or surgical care; the use of post-mortem fetal tissues for pharmacological and biochemical studies; and the participation of human fetuses in noninvasive investigations involving minimal or no risk. In addition, much valuable information was also obtained from research on animal fetuses as well as from studies of dead human fetuses.

Survey of the Literature - The Mahoney Report

In order to assess and define more accurately the role played by human fetal experimentation in the past, the National Commission for the Protection of Human Subjects of Biomedical and Behavioral Research contracted with Yale University (Dr. Maurice J. Mahoney being the principal investigator) to make an extensive literature survey based on a National Library MEDLARS search covering the indexing years 1969-74 and inclusive of January, 1975. The total number of citations was in excess of 3000 in a period which spanned approximately the last ten years.[1]

For purposes of convenience in summarizing this vast body of literature, Dr. Mahoney divided his report according to four general areas of investigation:

1. Normal and abnormal growth in development of the implanted fetus *in utero.*
2. Diagnosis of fetal disease or abnormality.
3. Fetal therapy and pharmacology.
4. Research with the previable fetus *ex utero.*

With respect to the first experimental group, over 600 publications were reviewed. Studies on the dead fetus provided much of the information regarding normal fetal growth. Investigations involving the fetus *in utero,* and organs and tissues removed from the dead fetus were employed to obtain information regarding fetal physiology.

To investigate fetal metabolic activity, some studies required the introduction of a chemical substance either directly into the fetal circulation or indirectly by administering it to the mother. Subsequently, the fetal umbilical cord blood was analyzed for the substance and/or for its metabolic products, or the tissues of the abortus were suitably examined for the appropriate substance.

The second group, a consideration of the diagnosis of fetal disease or abnormality, included some 1000 publications. Under this heading, Dr. Mahoney considered studies of: numerous genetic defects, Rh incompatibility between mother and fetus, neural tube defects, lung maturity, congenital heart disease and fetal well-being. To obtain the vast information included under these various headings, human fetuses were involved in a variety of procedures, among which were included: amniocentesis, fetography, diagnostic ultrasound and fetoscopy.

The third area of consideration was fetal therapy and pharmacology. Mahoney reported that out of more than 400 published studies, less than 80 involved pharmacological investigations requiring the use of living human fetuses. Of these latter studies, most were coincidental to clinically acceptable procedures. The drug studies included anesthetics and analgesics, cardiovascular agents, oxytoxic agents, hormones (such as oral contraceptives and insulin), anti-infective agents (such as antibiotics and anticonvulsants) and diuretics. These studies were generally retrospective and involved the fetus incidentally or after death. The techniques were, for the most part, non-invasive or at least placed the fetus at minimal risk. Some investigative studies, however, often prospective in nature, required the use of aborted fetuses whose tissues were analyzed for distribution and on whom metabolic studies of maternally administered drugs were done.

The fourth major category reviewed by Mahoney in his report dealt with research employing the nonviable fetus outside the uterus.[2] *This careful survey of the world literature identified less than 20 published articles in which the nonviable fetus was employed.* The only reported research efforts carried out in the United States on the living nonviable fetus *ex utero* (i.e., the nonviable premature infant in previous terminology) were those projects concerned with the development of an artificial life support system suitable for such infants. One study from the United States reported a technique by which the fetus, while still *in utero,* had his umbilical cord exposed and a drug injected into the umbilical vein. Afterward, the dead fetus was analyzed for the presence and distribution of the drug or its metabolites. Of the research done outside of the United States, the following may be cited as illustrative of a few studies:

1. Brain metabolism was isolated in eight human fetuses (a gestation age of 12-17 weeks) after hysterotomy abortion by perfusing the isolated head in order to determine whether the human fetal brain could metabolize ketone bodies (Finland).[3]
2. To determine innovative ways of supporting life in the fetus, eight fetuses (300-980 grams) obtained by hysterotomy abortion were immersed in a fluid and perfused with oxygenated blood through their umbilical vessels (England).[4]

In research of this nature on the living fetus not yet capable of maintaining vital functions independently, it is clear that the expected benefits of the research relate either to fetuses as a class or to an increase in biomedical knowledge in general rather than to the advantage of an individual fetus.

Definitions

As was mentioned, the Department of Health, Education and Welfare has published new rules and regulations governing fetal research. An understanding of the terminology employed in these regulations is necessary to a careful analysis of the issue of fetal experimentation. In order to identify the common and current nomenclature, the following definitions should be noted:

> "Pregnancy" encompasses the period of time from confirmation of implantation until expulsion or extraction of the fetus.
>
> "Fetus" means the product of conception from the time of implantation until a determination is made, following expulsion or extraction of the fetus, that it is viable.
>
> "Viable" as it pertains to the fetus means being able, after either spontaneous or induced delivery, to survive (given the benefit of available medical therapy) to the point of independently maintaining heart beat and respiration. The Secretary may, from time to time, taking into account medical advances, publish in the *Federal Register* guidelines to assist in determining whether a fetus is viable for purposes of this subpart. If a fetus is viable after delivery, it is a premature infant.
>
> "Nonviable fetus" means a fetus *ex utero* which, although living, is not viable.

> "Dead fetus" means a fetus *ex utero* which exhibits neither heart beat, spontaneous respiratory activity, spontaneous movement of voluntary muscles, nor pulsation of the umbilical cord (if still attached).[5]

Of specific concern in this report is that type of human fetal experimentation which has been called "non-therapeutic" research. However, there appears to be some ambiguity as to the meaning of that term. In their report to the Secretary of DHEW, the National Commission defined the two relevant terms "therapeutic" and "non-therapeutic" as follows:

> "Therapeutic research" refers to research designed to improve the health condition of the research subject by prophylactic, diagnostic or treatment methods that depart from standard medical practice but hold out a reasonable expectation of success.
>
> "Non-therapeutic research" refers to research not designed to improve the health condition of the research subject by prophylactic, diagnostic or treatment methods.[6]

To avoid any misunderstanding, it is appropriate to make explicit what is presumed in the term *non-therapeutic research,* the definition of which actually implies the following two elements:

1. No expected or intended benefit to the subject, which, in this case, would generally mean no improvement in the quantity or quality of life for the fetus who is the *subject* of the research.
2. There is an expectation of benefit, or at least intended, to others of that class, or to society at large, or to biomedical knowledge.[7]

The remainder of this study will now consider in depth the ethical challenges posed by the various types of fetal experimentation.

To conclude this section, the Commission's own summary of the Mahoney survey is concise:

> . . . research involving the fetus includes a broad spectrum of studies of the fetus both inside and outside the uterus. The research may be as innocuous as observation, or involve mild manipulation such as weighing or measuring, or more extensive manipulation such as altering the environment, administering a drug or agent, or noninvasive monitoring. Diagnostic studies may involve sampling amniotic fluid, urine, blood, or spinal fluid, or performing biopsies. The most extensive or invasive procedures include perfusion studies and other attempts to maintain function.[8]

Thus fetal experimentation in the past decade has ranged over a broad spectrum from minimal to rather extensive manipulation of living fetuses.

The Challenge of Ethical Concerns

It might be asked whether all or some of this information using human fetuses could have been obtained by means of animal experimentation. In response, it must be said that, while considerable contributions have been made with the use of animal fetuses, there are certain inherent limitations in the use of such fetuses to acquire knowledge about the anatomical, biochemical, and physiological development of the human fetus as well as to develop therapeutic procedures for human diseases. Because of the frequently unpredictable presence of marked interspecies differences in pharmacological response, the application to the human situation of information obtained from animal studies regarding drug toxicity, metabolism, and drug action requires great caution.

However, it should be emphasized that in animal experimentation the use of several different animal species will frequently help to avert disaster. The thalidomide incident is illustrative. If adequate preliminary toxicity studies had been done, the relatively slight toxic effects observable in the rat would have led to the use of the rhesus monkey, whose fetus demonstrates the same developmental anomalies as the human fetus.[9]

A recent report of the World Health Organization on fetal maturation recognized the past and continuing role of studies on experimental animals and advocated the use of a wider range of animal species in addition to the continued use of human fetal material "with due regard to ethical considerations."[10]

There is little question, nonetheless, that much of the actual research which led to the present state of fetology and perinatal medicine was derived from procedures that raised no major ethical questions. The problem began to arise partly as a consequence of the increasing availability of fetuses (perhaps related to the *Roe* v. *Wade* decision of the U.S. Supreme Court),[11] and partly due to the widening range of experimental procedures that could not directly benefit the fetal subjects, but which were viewed as possibly quickening the rate of medical progress in the area of fetology. It began to be anticipated that great strides in advancing scientific understanding of fetal development and in overcoming obstacles to respiratory adaptation to extra-uterine life could be made. Further, it was not merely the quest for new knowledge, as such, that raised questions, but also the use of certain proposed treatment procedures made possible by the availability of fetal material, such as, for example, transplantation of liver obtained from an aborted fetus for treatment of Fabry's disease.

Soon, however, critical questions began to emerge and disturb the conscience of the public as well as of the experimenters. What safeguards should be placed on fetal experimentation? Who can appropriately give consent for the fetus, especially when there is no intended or expected benefit for this fetus? Accordingly, the principal ethical questions might be stated thus:

1. Are there morally acceptable indications for involving live human fetuses in medical research for the purpose of advancing medical

knowledge and assuring the better health of future fetuses and infants, especially when such research may not be of benefit to those particular fetuses?

2. And if so, what would be appropriate regulations to govern such fetal research?

This study reflects on the above questions in light of secular and religious ethical traditions in order to discover guidelines consistent with Catholic belief and capable of commanding the broadest possible public support.

Summary

In the past decade, increasingly intensive research in neonatology and fetology has resulted in improved perinatal care. Much of this research on human fetuses, or the newborn, was done with a therapeutic intent and carried out in an ethically acceptable manner. A survey conducted by Dr. Maurice J. Mahoney of Yale University, at the request of the National Commission for the Protection of Human Subjects of Biomedical and Behavioral Research, reviewed some 3000 research papers and divided them into four different types of research protocols. According to Dr. Mahoney's analysis, only a very small percentage of these papers reported research that clearly was of a non-therapeutic nature and which involved more than minimal manipulation of the fetus. However, with the increased availability of human fetuses resulting from elective abortion, the ethical issues surrounding the employment of fetuses for medical research have become more acute and more urgently in demand for a solution.

CHAPTER I Footnotes

1. See *Federal Register,* "Protection of Human Subjects", 40(154):33532-33534, August 8, 1975. See also full report, March 14, 1975, submitted to the Commission.
2. Although the term "nonviable" will be used on occasion throughout this study, it should be recognized that it can be misleading if it is interpreted as providing an excuse for failing to make serious efforts to sustain the life of a premature infant.
3. Adam, P. A. J., Raiha, N., Rahiala, E. L., *et al:* "Cerebral Oxidation of Glucose and D-BOH-Butyrate by the Isolated Perfused Fetal Head", *Pediatric Research* 7: 309, 1973.
4. Chamberlain, G.: "An Artificial Placenta: The Development of an Extracorporeal System for Maintenance of Immature Infants with Respiratory Problems", *American Journal of Obstetrics and Gynecology* 100:615, 1968.
5. *Federal Register, op. cit.,* p. 33529.
6. *Ibid.,* p. 33532.
7. Although the definition as formulated by the Commission does not explicitly include the requirement that the research be of benefit to others, this element is explicitly mentioned throughout the document, e.g., *Deliberations* (B.2), (C.3) and *Recommendations* 4(a), 6(a), etc., in *op. cit.,* pp. 33545, 33547, 33548.
8. *Federal Register, op. cit.,* p. 33534.
9. Personal communication from Dr. Frances Kelsey (a FDA scientist whose vigilance prevented Thalidomide from reaching the United States market).
10. "Maturation of Fetal Body Systems", *World Health Organization Technical Report Series,* No. 540, p. 29, 1974.
11. *Roe vs. Wade,* 410 U.S. 113; 93 S. Ct. 705; 35 L. Ed. 2d 147 (1973).

2

Basic Human Rights and the Fetus in the Civic Community

Scientific research is a social activity which must be evaluated in terms of its social benefits and costs. While truth may be an absolute value, the process by which the advance of truth is achieved inevitably requires a degree of social control based on critical evaluation of the cost/benefit ratio.[1] This social dimension to research suggests that contemporary models of the civic community should be explored. Among the rights which result from being a citizen is the right to determine what will, or will not, be done to one's mental and physical being by others. Accordingly, the social controls for regulating the practice of experimentation with human subjects, first with reference to adults, then children, and, finally, the human fetus will be considered.

Human Rights in the Civic Community

Although human beings have lived in community from the beginning, the norms or morality by which they lived have sometimes been more the result of experience and intuition than of logical reflection. Yet, because human intuition requires rational elaboration, human beings have also attempted to articulate their moral norms and transmit them to successive generations in a coherent, systematic way.[2] Nations are considered "civilized" precisely to the degree that these articulated norms are designed to protect the rights of human beings as interrelated members of the human community, and to the degree that each individual is considered and treated as a *civis*.

The Basis of Human Rights

The very notion of "civilization" has advanced far beyond a simple opposite of "barbarism". In this twentieth century, it constitutes a world-view shared by most nations and expressed in the United Nations *Universal Declaration of Human Rights.*[3] This world-view affirms the value of human persons and proclaims the ethical will to overcome human suffering and to promote and protect the quality of human life. In spite of the tragic disasters of this century, advances in general knowledge, science, and technology do promise practical means to achieve these goals. However, this will be true only if this power is used in a truly civilized way, namely, to promote the rights of human beings in community, rather than to enslave them.[4]

Thus progress in civilization is a process by which the definition of the *civis* is more and more clearly articulated in terms of rights and duties. The right to vote was first extended in the United States from property-owners to all male whites, then to blacks, to women, and finally to eighteen-year-olds. At the same time, there has been increasing legislation to protect the rights of children, the aged, the insane, the helpless, those accused of crime, and even the condemned criminal. This extension has been based on the growing recognition of two facts: (1) Humanity forms a community in which a threat to the rights of one threatens the rights of all, and, (2) modern technology makes it possible for society to provide for needs of even its unproductive members. Although the present crisis of economic limits seems to weaken the force of the latter fact, it strengthens the former. The more the limits of world resources are realized, the more the interdependence of the entire human race is felt.[5]

However, this extension of civil rights by the State raises the question as to whether citizens, in fact, possess these rights as "inherent" or whether the State creates these rights at will. Certainly by recognizing and fostering such rights, the community does contribute to the humanness of developing human beings, but are these rights rooted in the individual or the community?

Collectivism vs. Individualism

One of the most evident features of the progress of civilization in the nineteenth and twentieth centuries has been the rise of collectivism and individualism as alternative explanations of the nature of human rights.[6]

Collectivist political philosophies, even those which are highly humanistic (as in the thought of Hegel and Marx), assert that human persons receive their very being from society and can assert no claim against the culture which has produced them, except on the grounds of the historical dialectic within the culture itself.[7] Thus, according to collectivist thought, a black person's right to freedom is not inherent in him as a person, but is appropriated to him by society at that point at which slavery is deemed socially obsolete.

This collectivism which dominates much of the world today has an alternate expression in the United States in the form of individualism. Individualism regards society as composed of politically relevant members viewed as abstract individuals who are the sole generators of their wants and the best judges of their own interests.[8] Criticized in France and moderated in England, individualism was celebrated in the United States as fostering those characteristics so necessary to the growth and prosperity of a new nation. Political individualism tended to be accompanied by an ethical individualism which "posits the individual man as the creator of whatever value can be wrested from an obscure universe."[9]

Individualism is seen as the polar opposite of collectivism, and this polarity is constantly exploited in the Cold War between the "free world" of individualism and the "communist world" of collectivism, with the "third world" of developing nations caught in between. However, this apparent opposition hides the fact that both views share a common rejection of faith in the *inherent* value of human beings. The collectivistic community assigns value to the individual on the basis of his or her social function, while the individualistic community recognizes the value only of those individuals who assert their own value competitively and establish it by productive performance or at least by their ability to impress the public or economically dominate it.

Collectivism may be regarded by some as socially destructive, but it has grown strong. Similarly in the United States, individualism seems to have succeeded. In the dynamics of social and political action in the history of this Republic, individualism and American social structures have effected mutual modifications and transformations, but the *ideals* of individualism are still present.[10]

Nor has the rise of the "counter-culture" in the 60's overcome this achievement-oriented individualism. It has only succeeded in giving individualism a new form —"privatism."[11] Many young people, while scorning "the establishment," seek only to find a way to live within the establishment economically, while keeping to themselves an area of private life in which they can exercise a still more intense individualism. This privatism has now been given legal recognition by the United States Supreme Court in its new doctrine of a "right to privacy" which tends to exempt from social concern and control all matters of human life which do not immediately interfere with public order and economic efficiency.[12]

It cannot be denied that in the United States, individualism has served in many ways to promote the growth of humanness for its citizens. Increased social and economic mobility, recognition of individual skills and abilities, and increased opportunities to exercise them, all can contribute to the growth of the individual as a human being. On the other hand, when status comes only through achievement, when society rewards those with ability and the individual becomes the bearer of his own worth on the basis of his productivity, what is the attitude of society toward those who cannot achieve, who are not socially productive, or who cannot seize power?[13]

The outcome of such individualism inevitably is *elitism* in which some of the best educated, the most wealthy and the most aggressive claim for their lifestyle a high "quality of life" and come to regard less successful human beings as a social burden.[14] At one level, this takes the form of an outcry against the unproductive poor, who have no function in this system, and who are seen as "welfare loafers."[15] At another, it becomes the "life-boat ethics" or "social triage," according to which the future ought to belong to well-born children in developed countries who alone have a chance for a life of high quality, while the "third world" and social outcasts are abandoned to their fate before they overwhelm the higher standard of living of the first and second worlds.[16] Finally, the result is the tendency of North Americans, so evident at recent world population conferences, to opt for those solutions to population overgrowth which depend primarily on contraception and abortion, rather than those that require radical economic and power readjustments.[17]

Speaking out of the models of the civic community just discussed, recently some ethicists have argued that a highly civilized community must simply draw a line beyond which it need not ascribe human rights to border-line humans, to those whose human functioning is very limited. They see this line-drawing not as an arbitrary restriction of human rights, but as a rational choice made in view of the legitimate purposes of human society. Thus the philosopher-physician H. Tristram Engelhardt, Jr., arguing from a Hegelian standpoint, attempts to show that society is justified both in imputing personhood to the infant and in refusing it to the unborn child. He believes that ontologically the infant is not yet a person, since it is still incapable of personal acts of reason and will. Nevertheless, unlike the unborn child, it can be treated *as if* it were a person because the mother, and others, relate to it in a personal manner.[18]

Similarly, another philosopher, Ronald M. Green, arguing from the viewpoint of recent ethicists in the tradition of British-American individualism stemming from Hobbes and Locke, arrives at much the same conclusions.[19] Green argues that the community is based on an implicit contract between competent adults from which arises a mutual obligation to acknowledge and defend the rights of these contracting parties. Hence only adults able to cooperate with the social system or to submit to it are persons in the strict sense. Children are treated as persons only because society is preparing them for adulthood. Defectives, the insane, the hopelessly ill, the senile are treated as persons only for the sake of competent adults, who otherwise would suffer sympathetically with them if they were neglected. However, since adults feel little sympathy with the unborn child, which is not yet capable of great or evident pain, it seems wise to Green that society not acknowledge the unborn as endowed with rights, because this would, without sufficient justification, restrict the rights of adults to be free of unwanted burdens.

Thus the arguments of Engelhardt and Green, startling in their line-drawing approach to subjects of human dignity, do reflect the common characteristic of collectivism and individualism, a rejection of inherent rights rooted within individual human beings. Thus both these contemporary models of the civic community seem to threaten the proper balance between the individual and the community which is the greatest achievement of civilization. Only by the establishment of a balance between collectivism and individualism can society discover a clear and unambiguous sense to the tradition of the rights of man embodied in the *Declaration of Independence,* the *United States Constitution* and the *United Nations Declaration of Human Rights,* all of which express the highest civic ideals of the United States and the world community.

The next chapter of this study will examine the basis of human rights in the personalist view which mediates between individualism and collectivism. The remainder of this chapter will unfold a reflective view of the way in which actual experience in the everyday life of a civilized community tends to support the rights of adults, children, and the unborn members of that community in the question of medical experimentation.

Social Controls for the Protection of Human Subjects in Experimentation

This reflection begins with the broader issue of medical experimentation on adult human beings. This is followed by considerations involved in experimentation on children and other dependent groups, and then, on the basis of generally accepted principles in these areas, the more specific and complex issue of fetal research within a civilized community will be discussed. Admittedly, this is to assume that the fetus is, in some sense, a "human being," although the fetus is not, by that very fact, being considered a "human person" with all the metaphysical and religious implications of that term.

Three basic presuppositions should be articulated. First, the terms "human being" and "human community" are strictly correlative, since neither is fully intelligible except in reference to the other. In Chapter III, this supposition will be discussed at length in order to bring out its full ontological implications. For the present it is sufficiently evident in a pragmatic sense. Obviously, human communities are composed of human beings and no human being can achieve a truly human life except as a member of one or more communities.

A second presupposition is that the human beings who constitute a community are *primarily* (though not exclusively) adults with a capacity for genuine interpersonal exchange with one another. This supposition is certainly debatable. But upon reflection, a third presupposition emerges, namely, that the adult members of the community bear the primary responsibility for their own survival as well as for the community's. Hence, of necessity the community is composed primarily of adults who are willing to accept responsibility for the survival of the community and who are able actually to effect it. Others may indeed belong to the community, who are not yet capable of assuming this responsibility, e.g., infants and children, or persons no longer capable of discharging such a responsibility, e.g., the infirm, the mentally defective. Provision for their survival should be made by the adult members of the community, for reasons to be mentioned below. But the life of the community here and now revolves around, and depends upon, the adult members.

Experimentation Involving Adults as Subjects

Given these presuppositions, what are the socially acceptable limits for medical experimentation on adult human beings, whether with or without their personal consent? Here there is not complete accord.[20] In all likelihood, most people would agree that an individual could knowingly and willingly submit to medical experimentation on himself if it were to benefit his own health. But it is not clear how many would approve human experimentation in cases where it contributes only to the health and well-being of others or to the advancement of medical knowledge at the expense of this human subject and without any benefit to him or her, even if the benefit to others is great. Although it may be granted that an informed, consenting adult may offer himself or herself as an experimental subject purely for the benefit of others, even with serious risk to life or health, still it is doubtful that such an act of self-sacrifice is ethical if death is the *probable* outcome of the experiment. Otherwise, the subject has equivalently been deprived of his or her life and hence of the capacity to be treated as a co-equal member of the community.

While animals may suitably be used for medical experimentation that usually involves the death of the "subject," it is generally held that human beings, to protect their own dignity as free and equal members of the community, should not, even by their own consent, subordinate themselves so completely to the will of other human beings. One might indeed argue that an individual who was already afflicted with a terminal illness (e.g., cancer) conceivably could submit to medical experiments even if death is known to be an early and likely consequence. But, even in this extreme case, the experimentation should be strictly limited to new techniques for combatting the disease in question. As Hans Jonas, the American philosopher, remarked, "Whatever the rights and wrongs of any experimentation on any patient—in the one case, at least that residue of identification is left him that it is his own affliction, his own kind of suffering which he helps to alleviate in others; and so in a sense, it is his own cause."[21]

Jonas makes an additional point: "What is wrong with making a person an experimental subject is not so much that we make him thereby a means (which happens in social contexts of all kinds), as that we make him a thing—a passive thing merely to be acted on."[22] For this same reason, most people would agree that medical experimentation performed on individuals either against their will or without their full consent (as may be the case in unrestricted experimentation with condemned criminals) is, as theologian Paul Ramsey suggests in a recent book, *The Ethics of Fetal Research,* "morally outrageous."[23] Individuals, to be sure, are conscripted for military service in order to defend their country against an aggressor. But this suspension of individual rights vis-a-vis the community's needs is generally regarded as legitimate only in a genuine emergency, when the survival both of the individual and of the community as a whole are at stake. Furthermore, conscripts are, or should be drafted not merely to be killed and expended as passive instruments, but are called as responsible and cooperative citizens to act in defense of the community of which they are members and whose benefits they have enjoyed and still hope to enjoy in the future. In the case of the subjugation of an unconsenting individual for experimentation, however, where the issue is not that of survival, but simply of progress in medical science, most contemporary ethicists would require that the individual's right to bodily integrity be strictly observed.

These general tenets which apply to human research are found concretized in two recent codes, *The Nuremburg Code* (1947) and *The Declaration of Helsinki* (1964), both of which were prompted largely by the medical atrocities uncovered in some of the Nazi concentration camps following World War II.[24] More recent are the guidelines promulgated in 1974 by the United States Department of Health, Education and Welfare to govern competent human adult research supported by that agency.[25] It was announced by the Department that further study was being conducted prior to publication of policies that would govern research involving pregnant women, children, fetuses, products of *in vitro* fertilization, prisoners and institutionalized mentally disabled individuals. Some of these have now been published and will be discussed in detail in Chapter VI. Inspection of all recent codes and regulations reveals that the obtaining of informed consent is absolutely essential to the conduct of human experimentation.

Experimentation Involving Children as Subjects

If the preceding remarks reflect currently acceptable general guidelines for adult members of the civilized community involved in human experimentation, what is to be said about those members of the community who either are not yet adults (infants, children) or who are not able to play an active role in the community (the infirm, the mentally defective, etc). Should there be different rules to govern medical experimentation on these other members? On the one hand, as noted above, the community is composed primarily of its adult members who bear the principal responsibility for its survival and continued well-being. On these grounds one might argue that, if medical experimentation on human subjects is to be permitted at all, it should be performed on those individuals who are least essential for the community's survival, that is, on those who are expendable.[26]

On the other hand, many, if not most adults would have serious misgivings about taking advantage of the weaker members of the community, even if it is done in the interests of medical science. The very condition of being weak or helpless elicits from the stronger, adult members of the civilized community increased concern that they do not suffer more intensely as a consequence. To quote Hans Jonas once again, "utter helplessness demands utter protection."[27] Yet, there are those who might ask whether this sentiment of compassion for the weak is grounded in a truly reasonable attitude of the adult members of the community? Or is it rather, as some believe, a form of sentimentality which ought to be curtailed in favor of a recognized higher good, namely progress in medical science, and with it, the increased well-being of the community as a whole.

No universally acceptable answer can be given to this question since we are dealing here with a primitive moral judgment which arises primarily, not out of logical argumentation or philosophical reflection, but out of past experience and moral intuition. Yet it can be forcefully urged against a purely utilitarian approach to medical experimentation that the adult community, in sacrificing its weaker members to the goal of increased medical technology, would be actually embarking upon a course of self-destruction. Because of the inherent interdependence of its members, genuine community can perdure only in virtue of the respect and concern which the members have for one another. When the primary civil rights of the weaker members of the community, however, are deliberately discarded by the stronger members for strictly pragmatic reasons, then there is no compelling reason for these same stronger members of the community still to relate to one another in a civilized way. Community life is then openly based on utilitarian values and on the power of its stronger members. As the community progressively restricts the primary rights of its weaker members it becomes progressively less human and less civilized, because distinctive human values are no longer operative.[28]

Consequently, the adult members of the community, in protecting the primary human rights of the weak and powerless in their midst, are actually expressing to one another the moral equality of their common humanity, regardless of inequality in strength, health, and physical development. This is the basis of their own life in community with one another. The primary human rights are the bases of civil rights and civilization itself. Because of this element human communities are distinguished from animal "communities." Hence, the decision to use the same rules *(mutatis mutandis)* for medical experimentation upon children, the infirm, the mentally defective, etc., as for research upon healthy adult members of the community is actually a form of self-protection for the community as a whole. It is a decision rooted in the actual relationships found in a civilized community. It should be noted that the elitist form of individualism and the totalitarian collectivism discussed earlier in this chapter as contemporary models of the civic community, more easily tend to compromise the rights of these weaker members of the community.

Experimentation Involving Fetuses as Subjects

At this point what can be said about fetal experimentation? Fetuses will here be considered as "human beings" in order to avoid the philosophical and theological commitment involved in giving them the status of "human persons." Despite their considerable dependence upon a maternal womb, they are biologically established as new and separate individual beings. They are genetically unique and are already launched in the process of human development which continues until death. Fetal life is human life, albeit in its incipient stages. As Dr. Bernard N. Nathanson, former director of an abortion clinic in New York, notes, "Life is an interdependent phenomenon for us all. It is a continuous spectrum that begins *in utero* and ends in death—the bands of the spectrum are designated by words such as fetus, infant, child, adolescent, and adult."[29] Hence, experimentation on fetuses *is* experimentation on human beings, even though the human beings in question may not yet be considered persons in the legal, psychological, or sociological senses of that word.[30]

A fetus lives a hidden life, invisible to the community, yet if the fetus is truly a "human subject" rather than a mere "object" or "thing" it must be treated as a human being and hence is under the protection of the same rules for human experimentation as other members of a civilized human community. Such a community will not permit its stronger adult members to victimize children or other weaker members. Must it not afford the same protection for human subjects at the fetal stage of development?

The danger, noted above, that the adult members of the community might lose all respect for each other's rights, as a result of ethically questionable medical practices, would seem to be just as evident in uninhibited experimentation on fetuses as in experimentation on children, the infirm, the mentally defective, etc. Fetuses are not fully free and independent, but neither are these other groups. A living human being in any stage of development has to be treated as precious, or it will soon be callously abused.

At the same time, fetuses should not be over-protected, i.e., spared from experimentation which would benefit them and which would be permissible in analogous cases of children or adults unable to give consent. Proxy consent for therapeutic or minimal risk non-therapeutic experimentation with subjects who are children, mentally handicapped, unconscious, etc. is normally obtained from parents or guardians. It would seem that in this respect the fetus does not constitute a special category, but should be protected as well by whatever rules are applicable to adults and children.

The above reflection about the actual experience of civilized communities suggests the necessity of recognizing the primary rights of even the weakest members for the good of the whole community. Virtually unrestricted experimentation on human fetuses would set a dangerous precedent of subordinating individuals (or whole classes of individuals) to the presumed interests of the community as a whole. A risk/benefit estimate in medical procedures normally applies to the risk and benefit of the same individual. If, however, the life and well-being of fetuses can be risked for the benefit of the rest of the community, then what is to prevent application of the same procedure to still other groups of individuals within the community at other stages of development: e.g., infants and children, the retarded and handicapped, the senile? This would typify the "might makes right" ideology of rugged individualism or the exploitation of individuals by the collectivist community.

Impact of the Supreme Court Decision on Fetal Experimentation

Admittedly, the recent *Roe* v. *Wade* decision of the United States Supreme Court opened the door to a practice that could lead potentially to relatively unlimited fetal experimentation in this country. In effect, the Supreme Court said in that decision that it need not resolve the difficult question of when full human life begins. It then decided that individual states may not make laws to limit abortions except in the last trimester. Thus, without resolving the doubt about fetal status, the Court made great concessions to the mother in a potential conflict of interest with her fetus. Using the same logic, the Court might also overthrow federal or state laws forbidding non-therapeutic fetal experimentation. That is, if within certain limits, the mother's personal preferences already take precedence over the life of the individual fetus, then it might be asked why should not the welfare of whole groups of future human beings be allowed to take precedence over the life of individual fetuses selected for experimentation? Thus the Supreme Court would complement the privatism of *Roe* v. *Wade,* where a mother's right to privacy was the operative factor, with a collective discrimination, where fetuses are exploited by the class of individuals with power. The step would be from *rejection* of the fetus in an individual conflict case to *subjection* of the fetus to the needs of medical research and the common good of society.

Of course, this particular possibility at the present time, is pure speculation, pending further action by the United States Supreme Court. It offers a dramatic illustration, however, of the fact that, without carefully specified controls, unlimited fetal experimentation poses a threat, not only to fetuses, but to the civilized community as a whole. The precedent of subordinating the most helpless and least developed members of the community to the advantages of others, even to other future members of the same class, might well reverse the flow of community concern for civil rights and civil liberties. If so, then unrestricted fetal experimentation would, in the long run, significantly decivilize the human community.

Summary

Human beings have lived in some kind of community from the earliest ages of their existence on earth. Through the United Nations' Universal

Declaration of Human Rights, the human community has expressed the ethical will to promote the quality of human life. Based on the realization that a threat to the rights of one is implicitly a threat to the rights of all, there has been, generally, increasing legislation to protect the rights of the children, the aged, the insane, and the helpless.

But the *source* of these rights for which the community expresses concern is extrinsic to the individual in two prominent models of the civic community. Collectivism traces the value of the individual to the community's recognition of his or her social function. According to the tenets of individualism, the human being must be able to establish his or her value by productive performance. In neither case is it granted that the human being has an inherent, intrinsic value independently of the community's attribution of such value.

However, a reflection upon the actual experience of civilized communities suggests the necessity of recognizing the primary rights of even the weakest members. For example, the *Nuremberg Code* and the *Declaration of Helsinki,* resulting from the experience of the Nazi atrocities, clearly provide for informed consent as an absolute prerequisite for the participation of adult subjects in experimentation. With regard to the involvement of children in medical research, most adults would be very reluctant to take advantage of the weaker members of the human community, even if it be for the improvement of the health of future children. This attitude reflects the basic equality of all humans in spite of inequality in secondary characteristics. Hence, because fetuses are truly human *subjects* rather than merely *objects,* their very helplessness seems to demand all the more that they be protected by the stronger, adult members of the community.

Virtually unrestricted experimentation on human subjects would set a dangerous precedent of subordinating individuals to the benefit of the community as a whole. Even the *Roe v. Wade* abortion decision limits abortion to cases of conflict of the fetus with the mother and does not subject the fetus to the needs or demands of society as a whole. Nonetheless, carefully designed controls have become necessary, not only for the protection of the fetus, but indirectly for the future well-being of the entire human community.

CHAPTER II Footnotes

1. At this point we can assume as a least common denominator of ethical discussion a cost/benefit or utilitarian point of view. In Chapter III we attempt to establish the human person as an end in itself.
2. See Edel, Mary and Abraham, *Anthropology and Ethics,* Cleveland Case Western Reserve University, 1968, especially Chapter IV, "On Being a Good Mother" (pp. 39 ff.) for a discussion of the way anthropology deals with the modes by which moral standards are constituted in different cultures.
3. "Whereas recognition of the inherent dignity and of the equal and inalienable rights of all members of the human family is the foundation of freedom, justice and peace in the world . . ." Preamble of the *Universal Declaration of Human Rights.* Note the terms "inherent" and "inalienable." This is not merely an abstract ideal, because the

Declaration was the direct outcome of the historic experience of World War II, as the rest of the Preamble implies. The World Synod of Catholic Bishops declared on December 9, 1971 in their document *Justice in the World,* "Never before have the forces working for bringing about a unified world society appeared so powerful and dynamic; they are rooted in the awareness of the full basic equality as well as the human dignity of all. Since men are members of the same human family, they are indissolubly linked with one another in the one destiny of the world, in the responsibility for which they all share."

4. See Beard, Charles A. and Mary, *The Rise of American Civilization,* vol. iv of *The American Spirit,* New York: The MacMillan Co., 1942, pp. 1-97.
5. Thus the Stockholm Conference on the Human Environment, sponsored in 1972 by the United Nations, adopted 26 principles based on the necessity of international cooperation in view of economic limits. For discussion, see Francis, John, "Ethics of Natural Resource Use", *Anticipation* 17:19-30, May, 1974, published by Church and Society, World Council of Churches, Geneva.
6. See Lukes, Steven, *Individualism,* Oxford: Basil Blackwell, 1973, p.79.
7. See Fromm, Eric, *Marx's Concept of Man,* New York: F. Unger, 1961 and Kamenka, Eugene, *The Ethical Foundations of Marxism,* New York: Praeger, 1962.
8. See Lukes, *loc. cit.*
9. Steinfels, Peter, "Individualism: No Exit", *The Hastings Center Studies,* II, September, 1974, p. 21.
10. "The three cardinal values of the Objectivist ethics—the three values which together, are the means to and realization of one's ultimate value, one's own life—are: Reason, Purpose, Self-Esteem, with their three corresponding virtues: Rationality, Productiveness, Pride. Productive work is the central *purpose* of a rational man's life, the central value that integrates and determines the hierarchy of all his other values. Reason is the source, the precondition of his productive work—pride is the result." Rand, Ayn, *The Virtue of Selfishness,* New York: Signet Books, New American Library, 1964. Rand sets up a false dichotomy between Selfishness and Altruism and between Reason and Mysticism.
11. "A third split in the new culture (the "counter-culture") is the conflict between individualism and collectivism. On this question the new culture talks out of both sides of its mouth, one moment putting ideals of cooperation and community against old-culture competitiveness, the next moment espousing the old culture in its most extreme form with exhortations to "do your thing". . . This problem is rarely faced honestly by new-culture adherents, who seem unaware of the conservatism involved in their attachment to individualistic principles." Statler, Philip E., "Cultures in Collision", (an excerpt from his *The Pursuit of Loneliness,* Boston: Beacon Press, 1970) *Psychology Today,* July, 1970, p. 68.
12. See Weddington, S. R., "Woman's Right of Privacy", *Perkins Journal of Theology* 27:35-41, Fall, 1973 for a discussion of the right of privacy as it is now being interpreted. Ms. Weddington was the lawyer who developed this doctrine before the Supreme Court in the abortion case *Roe v. Wade.*
13. Ward, John William, "Individualism: Ideology or Utopia?", *Hastings Center Studies* II, September, 1974, p. 7.
14. Goulet, Denis, "Christian Ethics and World Development: A Critical Perspective", an as yet unpublished address delivered at the 15th Annual Meeting of the American Society of Christian Ethics, January 18-20, 1974 in Chicago. Goulet showed that the Third World rightly resents the way the dominant societies seek to push a population control policy on them as the solution of the world crisis of economic limits. The only solution, Goulet argues, is an overarching network of incentives and motivations which can activate the entire social order in underdeveloped countries. The dominant countries seek to cover over this fact because it raises the fundamental issue of a world economic order founded on profit for the richest and strongest.
15. For a careful refutation of these myths see *Poverty in American Democracy: A Study of Social Power,* Campaign for Human Development, United States Catholic Conference, Washington, D.C., 1974.
16. See Hardin, G., "Living on a Lifeboat", *Psychology Today* 8:7-12, December, 1974.
17. See McLaughlin, Martin M., "Food for the World", *Commonweal,* December 20, 1974, 2666-69; and Blewett, Jane W., "System in Crisis: Rome Food Conference", *America*

132:144-149, March, 1975.

18. See Engelhardt,Tristram,Jr., "Viability, Abortion, and the Difference between a Fetus and an Infant", *American Journal of Obstetrics and Gynecology* 116:429-434, June 1, 1973; also "Beginnings of Personhood: Philosophical Considerations", Perkins Journal of Theology 27:2, Fall, 1973.
19. Green, Ronald M., "Conferred Rights and the Fetus", *Journal of Religious Ethics* 2:55-83, Spring, 1974; see also "Abortion and Promise-Keeping", *Christianity and Crisis* 27:109-113, May 15, 1967.
20. See Freund, Paul A., "Introduction to the Issue 'Ethical Aspects of Experimentation with Human Subjects'", *Daedalus* XCVIII, 1969, p. viii-viv.
21. Jonas, Hans, "Philosophical Reflections on Experimenting with Human Subjects", *Daedalus* XCVIII, 1969, p. 243.
22. *Ibid.,* p. 235. Perhaps it would be better to say, "It is never permitted to make a person a *mere* means", i.e., to ignore that a person, as a totality, is *always* an end, although he or she may be regarded or used as a means in some partial respect.
23. Ramsey, Paul, *The Ethics of Fetal Research,* New Haven: Yale University Press, 1975, p. 33.
24. A brief but excellent review of the early post-war efforts to formulate some practical rules to govern human experimentation may be found in an article by Beecher, Henry K., "Experimentation in Man", *Journal of the American Medical Association* 169(5):109-126, January 31, 1959.
25. *Federal Register* 39(105):18914-18920, May 30, 1974.
26. Obviously, children are, from another point of view, *indispensable* for the survival of the community. But potentially lethal experimentation on *some* infants or young children would not seem to pose as serious a threat as similar experimentation on the adult leaders of the community.
27. Jonas, *op.cit.,* p. 240.
28. Thus the Dred Scott decision of the United States Supreme Court on March 6, 1857, which categorized Negroes legally as non-persons is generally accepted today as a regressive step in American civilization. Nonetheless, it might be argued by some that too much concern about survival of the weaker members might be injurious to the well-being of the community by reducing its over-all effectiveness in a highly competitive, intercommunity environment.
29. Nathanson, Dr. Bernard N., "Deeper Into Abortion", *The New England Journal of Medicine,* November 28, 1974.
30. There is good reason to consider fetuses to be human persons in the existential or ontological sense of that word. See Chapter III of this Study for a more detailed discussion of this point.

3

Human Personhood and the Fetus in the Personalist Community

The organization of human beings into the civic community discussed above seems to emerge from the needs that humans experience to relate to one another and cooperate for their mutual benefit. Life in community, therefore, can be viewed as being just as natural a need for humans as the need for food and shelter. "Man's corporate life does not run along tracks that are directed by instinct and fixed by heredity," says the German theologian Wolfhart Pannenberg.[1] "Neither do its forms emerge from arbitrary agreements between individuals, so that they would be inconsequential for our humanity. Rather, they are invented because everything in man is aimed at community with others."[2] Consequently, this chapter will transcend the pragmatic and legal considerations dealt with in Chapter II to a deeper philosophical analysis of human dignity and personhood.

The Personalist Community

Humanists, generally, whether theistic or non-theistic, have recognized the interpersonal character of human experience. For instance, the "Paris Statement of 1966" written by a prominent group of secular humanists, noted that, "Man becomes human in society; society should provide conditions for the fullest possible development of each man."[3] Another proposition from that same statement affirmed "the unity of man and a common responsibility of all men for all men."[4]

The community of individuals who participate in a common life as freely developing and mutually interacting members can be described as a *personalist* or *person-centered* community. The Vatican Council's document, *Pastoral Constitution on the Church in the Modern World,* reflects this developmental approach to life in society: "Man's social nature makes it evident that the progress of the human person and the advance of society itself hinge on each other. From the beginning, the subject and the goal of all social institutions is and must be the human person, which, for its part, and by its very nature, stands completely in need of social life."[5]

Thus, an inquiry into the personhood of the fetus might profitably uncover the direction of a more progressive civilization, wherein greater dignity is conferred on the individual person. However, that question has an antecedent query which is usually not articulated: Do adults *want* to include or exclude the fetus in the class of persons?[6] One group, including those under the pressure of problems resulting from unwanted pregnancies, defective children, economic considerations, maternal well-being, as well as those who strongly believe that significant improvement in health care might be made through certain types of fetal experimentation desire that the fetus not be given the attribute of personhood. Another group of the opposite persuasion, who, although neither unaware of, nor insensitive to, those agonizing problems, feel constrained in conscience by the pressure of their concern for moral consistency in their understanding and application of human values to include the fetus in the category of persons. Consequently, the former will tend to formulate a definition of person that will exclude the fetus, while the latter will arrive at a definition in which the fetus would be included.

The inquiry here will attempt to decide whether or not the fetus should be included in the definition of *person* by first asking what is a person in those instances where there is no dispute (e.g., an awake, alert and normal adult), and then, secondly, looking at the difficult case of the fetus to see if the fetus is a person in any sense. A third analysis will then ask if the adult community should protect the fetus as a person, and the final brief discussion will consider the attitudes of a person-centered community toward the fetus as a basis for the subsequent development of guidelines for fetal experimentation.

Characteristics of the Human Person

Alexander Solzhenitsyn, the Russian Nobel Laureate, has written: "The meaning of existence (is) to preserve unspoiled, undisturbed, and undistorted the image of eternity with which each person is born."[7] Human beings have discovered that man "is not merely an instance of the universal, each man is something unique."[8]

Genetic discoveries of recent decades further reinforce the idea of the uniqueness of the individual: The combination of genes which each person receives from his parents is utterly individualized. Even identical (monozygotic) twins, who presumably share identical nuclear genes, demonstrate some individuation, sometimes subtle, but nonetheless, real.[9] This uniqueness and un-repeatability of each human person renders unsatisfactory all attempts to *define* personhood adequately. It does suggest that human personhood is a lived mystery, a profound mystery, a fullness and richness of corporeal existence. Human persons, to be sure, can be described in terms of their role before the law, but this is a *legal* definition of personhood which does not touch the core of the "mystery of man."

Any description of person emerging from a consideration of undisputed examples of persons will build upon the conscious awareness of freedom, i.e., the power of self-determination. To be a person is to be free, with all the creative and transcending capacities of a rational nature at one's disposal.

In contrast to human behavior is that determinism which characterizes the higher primates such as the chimpanzee or the gorilla. Washoe, the chimpanzee who was taught to communicate in the American sign language, and Sarah, another chimpanzee who had a reading and writing vocabulary of some 130 "words" based on variously shaped and colored plastic pieces, for example, are likewise each a "living substance."[10] But these chimpanzees are not free—virtually nothing remains for their future but the natural developmental unfolding of chimpanzee life when left to themselves. However, they, as so many other animals—dogs, parrots, seals, fish—can be taught by man to perform according to certain behavior patterns not found in the wild, but they are still severely limited by their physical structure and especially by their central nervous system. Chimpanzees, for example, apart from other reasons, cannot learn to speak because they lack the appropriate anatomical structures for human-type speech.

A human being, on the other hand, is radically free; he or she is a living act of self-determination.[11] Whatever may have been the historical origin of humankind (evolutionary or special creation) there is no evidence that the tremendous human cultural development was due to the instructions received from a member of an alien and superior species (UFO's notwithstanding!). This creative capacity is one expression of man's freedom. Thus, to be a person means to be called to become more and more human through rational effort, to live a life of genuine self-possession. The human being, to be sure, is rooted in physical nature by bodily being and is directed to nature with his or her whole activity. But, to be a human being, by reason of personhood, is to possess a living and creative freedom, which transforms both nature at large and his or her own nature by means of culture. Thus even theistic philosophers who believe in God as Creator can still say with atheistic thinkers that the human person is self-creative.

Persons, however, cannot develop their freedom in a social vacuum. Father Martin D'Arcy, the British theologian, describes how human persons "first discover others and salute them and address them as persons, as beings and persons who are most decidedly not ourselves, who demand of us that we treat them as beings who possess their own inalienable individuality and perfection."[12] Human persons are, accordingly, "present" to one another, and this "presence" manifests the essentially relational dimension of personhood.

In developing self-consciousness the reflection which discloses the self has already also disclosed the "thou," for the self of human experience is an "I" only in the face of a "thou." Seen in this light, *personhood is correlative to community,* even a community composed of just two individuals. However, it seems that a larger number of individuals are required to provide those variations of personal interaction necessary for a full development of the person. That is, the community exists in virtue of the persons; but the persons themselves can achieve full expression of personhood only in and through the life of the community.

The relations of persons seem to transcend the physical order of nature, especially, in its temporal aspects. The following remark of the personalist philosopher, Gabriel Marcel, is apropos: "To love a person is to say to him, 'Thou at least shalt not die.'"[13] Marcel sees this kind of statement as a translation into language of the experience of "presence" in which persons reach beyond the limits of the world of things and objects. "We must maintain that insofar as we are not things, insofar as we refuse to allow ourselves to be reduced to the condition of things, we belong to an entirely different world-dimension, and it is this dimension which can and must be called supra-temporal."[14]

Definitions of Personhood

Scholastic philosophy described the corporeal continuity of a living being with the aid of its concept of a "living substance." The life process continually changes and renews the physical cells of a living substance but the "substantial form" provides for continuity and specificity for that individual. The early sixth century philosopher Boethius said, for example, that a person is an "individual substance of a rational nature."[15] Unfortunately, such language does not adequately express the dynamic quality of self-creative growth and spiritual achievement which sets the human "individual substance" above and beyond any other apparent "living substance" known to man. But it does emphasize that *personhood belongs to each human being from the core of his or her being; it is an endowment, not an achievement, of human nature.* In a similar vein, Thomas Aquinas understood personhood to imply a *complete* substance, *subsisting* by itself, and *distinguished* from all others.[16] Such scholastic descriptions suggest the profound difference between a person and the whole remaining world of visible creation. The person enjoys complete substantiality and lives out the projections of his or her own will in a way unmatched among animals or other living substances.

Admittedly the scholastic perspective which defined persons in the context of the subsistent unity of matter and form is not the perspective of modern personalists like Marcel. But both positions share common insights about the metaphysical unity and continuity of human persons. According to both positions, personhood must ultimately be assessed in terms of a unique mode of being and existing, rather than of acting, which is dependent upon the former.

This basic conviction, that personhood is a special kind of being, provides a basis for the familiar principle in ethics and politics of the "moral equality of all persons." In fact, it seems difficult to defend adequately such equality on grounds less intrinsic to the person, grounds such as social acceptance or social agreement. These grounds may serve conveniently as criteria for a sociological description of personhood, but not for the moral *equality* of all persons. Without committing itself to a philosophical criterion of personhood, an important consensus statement signed by 200 humanists, called the *Humanist Manifesto II* of 1973, clearly accepted the principle of the moral equality of all persons and opposed "all discrimination based upon race, religion, sex, age or national origin."[17] This document voiced concern for "the welfare of the aged, the infirm, the disadvantaged, and also for the outcasts—the mentally retarded, abandoned or abused children, the handicapped, prisoners, and addicts—for *all* who are neglected or ignored by society."

However, it is not self-evident that these reflections on human personhood apply to the human fetus in all stages or to any stage of gestation. Thus the second question must be asked: Is the fetus a person in any sense?

The Fetus and Personhood

Inadequacy of Legal and Pychological Criteria.

This question cannot be answered merely in a legal sense. The present legal status of the fetus seems to depend on whether it is inside or outside the womb of the mother. While the recent Supreme Court decision of *Roe* v. *Wade* seriously impugned the legal status of the fetus, the more recent Edelin case was an indication, on the other hand, of the law's concern for the fetus outside the mother or at least once the process of removal had begun. In any case, legal definitions of personhood represent constructions of the law rather than reflections of a philosophical understanding of personhood itself.

Nor can the above question be considered merely in a psychological sense. The strict psychological description of a human person concentrates upon the evidence of uniquely personal functions. Common sense indicates that human persons can *be* persons without actively functioning for example, as in sleep. Limiting the discussion of personhood only to those persons actively and actually functioning in personal relationships denies personhood not only to sleeping people, but to the insane, the unconscious, the dying, and the newborn infants. "To *be* a person means more than to *function* as a person. Function ultimately results from structure, and structure is operative long before functions appear."[18]

Deciding who is a person thus becomes a question to be resolved not only by psychological criteria or legal definitions, but also by philosophical examination and interdisciplinary reflection. To pose the question, "Is the fetus a human person?" means to ask an ontological question about a living human being. That is, apart from the usual external manifestations of personhood, can the human fetus properly be denominated a "person" due to a mode of its existence by the reality intrinsic to it? As Engelhardt states, (see p.28), "Is the fetus merely an animal with the potential of becoming more?" Or is the fetus existentially already a person in some primordial sense?"

Biological Criteria and Fetal Personhood

It will be necessary to define and/or describe the fetus itself, according to biological criteria. The Mahoney Report used as a working definition of *fetus* the following: "The human embryo from conception to delivery, without distinction of an embryonic and fetal period."[19] However, the National Commission for the Protection of Human Subjects of Biomedical and Behavioral Research, in their published statement, defined the fetus as "the human from the time of implantation until a determination is made following delivery that it is viable or possibly viable. If it is viable or possibly viable, it is thereupon designated an infant."[20] By the latter definition, if it is not viable or even possibly so, even though momentarily alive, it remains classified as a fetus.

Neither of these definitions convey adequately the living reality of the fetus. A more descriptive statement is found in an article by the New Zealand obstetrician A. W. Liley, "The Foetus as Personality." In part this reads as follows:

> Far from being an inert passenger in a pregnant mother, the foetus is very much in command of the pregnancy. . . . It is the foetus who determines the duration of pregnancy. . . . who decides which way he will lie in pregnancy and which way he will present in labour. . . . The foetus is in neither stupor nor hypoxic coma. . . . Foetal comfort determines foetal position. The foetus is responsive to pressure and touch. . . . flashing lights applied to the maternal abdominal wall produced fluctuations in foetal heart rate. . . . Sudden noise in a quiet room. . . . startles the foetus. . . .[21]

Obviously most of these fetal activities are possible only after some degree of fetal development. But the *capacity* to respond thus, and the capacity to be a human infant, child, adolescent, adult is already programmed in the zygote, primarily coded in the 23 pairs of chromosomes. The fetus from its inception shows a gradual growth and differentiation without any significant discontinuities until the death of the individual. Thus the human fetus shows itself as an organism with an inner dynamism which, apart from accident or defect, naturally leads it to full adulthood in a smooth progression. Gradually, characteristics are manifested, which, in their later developed state, will distinguish the fetus as an *adult* person.

Should however this developing fetus be considered a human person from the moment of conception? Many recent writers try to avoid this question by rejecting static, absolute conceptions about the origin of personhood, in favor of more dynamic terms in reference to the "process" by which the fetus gradually develops into a human person. This issue will now be discussed in two stages: a) Personhood as Process and b) Delayed Hominization.

Fetal Development and Personhood as Process. Undoubtedly, all thinking about living beings should always be process-oriented since organic life exists only in process. However, the slightest reflection shows that unless the life process of a living being is conceived as one homogeneous movement taking place in a single organism, one must not only talk of *the* "life-process" but of many distinct processes, and of many individual organisms, each of which has its own individual, empirically identifiable life process. *This* individual living being may be only a moment in the history of the evolution of life, but nevertheless it is an individual, which began to exist at some point in time, and will cease to exist at another.

Therefore, in regard to an individual person, one must ask: When did *this* person begin, and, when did his or her biography end? At what point in time did this person emerge as a distinct individual having his or her life process to live out? If this moment is later than conception, then there should be some empirical evidence of an actual time, a threshold at which this human person begins to exist.[22] Efforts to pinpoint such an exact time (implantation, viability, birth, socialization), as will be argued below, do not stand up under examination. It is very difficult to conceive how an individual human organism already in existence and already in the process of individual development, can at a subsequent point of time *become* a person. As the eminent Methodist theologian Albert Outler has said, "Personhood is not a *part* of the human organism, nor is it inserted into a process of organic development at some magic moment. It *is* the human organism oriented towards its transcendental matrix, in which it lives and moves and has its being."[23]

On the other hand, if one decides that human personhood begins at conception, this requires the acceptance of the idea of a person who is a single, minute cell. At first glance, it seems preposterous to believe that the almost infinitely complex system which constitutes a human personality could be present in such a tiny bit of protoplasm, yet this is what is implied. As the Jesuit theologian Joseph Mangan has said, "It would be incorrect to refer to the human body as being only virtually or potentially present in the zygote. The human body is *actually* present, the *adult* human body is potentially present."[24] Paul Ramsey also says, "In a remarkable way, modern genetics also teaches there are 'formal causes,' immanent principles, or constitutive elements long before there is any shape or motion or discernible size."[25]

Yet, this seemingly incredible assertion becomes more plausible by fully rejecting the Cartesian dualism of "body" and "mind." If the human person is actually a body-mind unity, then there is nothing unreasonable in believing that as the human body develops out of a single cell as a continuous organism, so human personhood develops out of a single cell as a continuous, unique individuality. As Emmanuel Mounier, a leader in personalist thinking, has said, "I am a person from my elementary existence upward, and my embodied existence, far from depersonalizing me, is a factor essential to my personal status."[26] Or as philosopher Louis Dupré says: "Although personhood is essentially a dynamic entity not fully realized even at life's peak, it must nevertheless be minimally present already at life's humble beginnings."[27]

Moreover, science today has made familiar two concepts, "system" and "information," which can assist this analysis. Any organism is a system, a stable structure that perdures through countless changes of the actual matter out of which the system is composed. The matter in a human body changes many times during life, the "I" as a unique and individual system continues through all these changes. A living system, furthermore, is one which develops and differentiates its parts, while remaining essentially the same unit. Thus the adult person is a highly developed and differentiated complex which has unfolded from a much less differentiated whole, but the adult, nonetheless, is still the *same* system.

How is this possible? It is here that the concept of "information" is relevant. The adult organism is not identical with the primordial organism as if it were simply an enlargement, an expanded or blown-up version of miniature. That notion is "preformism," a type of embryology long ago abandoned by scientists. Rather this identity is established by the fact that in the primordial organism there is the "information" or code specifying the *relations* (both static and dynamic) which will determine the adult structure and the entire sequence of differentiating events necessary to its development.

However, some writers argue that conception itself is only one moment in a much longer process. Why not say that the person is already present in the sperm or ovum, or that this person was potentially present at the very beginning of evolution when life began on the planet? Is it not arbitrary to pick out some one moment in this continuous process? "Human life is an unbroken continuum extending from one person to another," writes the philosopher-physician H. Tristram Engelhardt.[29] Such authors may also object that the zygote is only *potentially* a human person, and this potentiality for the emergence of this or that person has always been present in the very fact of the existence of life on earth. Dr. Engelhardt, in another article, wrote:

> . . . one can value potential but yet unborn persons, anxiously awaited children, protended grandchildren, future generations for whom one may tend the earth with care. But again, it is values, not rights, which guide these attitudes.
>
> Even the more concrete potentiality of the fetus is not yet the potentiality of anyone—there is not yet a "who" present whose poten-

tiality it is. There is not yet a "who" to have personal rights. Rather, the fetus' value is in terms of its promise of, or potentiality for becoming a person. But the fetus is not yet valuable to itself but to others for whom it has value; the fetus is not yet a person to whom things have value. That is, the value of the fetus is implicit in the fetus, and for others, but not for itself. The fetus does not yet have value in and for itself.[30]

On the other hand, others see the fetus as an *actual* human being and do not see much significance in an attempt to distinguish between a "human being" and a "human person." Thus Helmut Thielicke, the Protestant ethicist, writes, "For once impregnation has taken place, it is no longer a question of whether the persons concerned have responsibility for a *possible* parenthood; they have *become parents.*"[31] And Dupré writes, "What we find before functional personhood is that dynamic combination of presence and absence moving toward ever greater presence to which the ancients attributed the name of potency."[32] Thus it is obvious that much of the controversy and confusion on this whole question is due to philosophical equivocations about the various meanings of "actuality" and "potentiality."

In striving for greater clarity in this matter one must first distinguish between the "potential" and the "possible." "Future generations" are mere possibilities. The ovum and the sperm, however, are actual entities, with the active potency or capacity to produce a new organism through fusion. However, they are not themselves the new, independent organism, and as long as they remain separated, the new organism remains a mere possibility. Thus future generations, and ova and sperm-cells are not persons and do not have human rights.

The zygote, however, is an independent organism, an *actual* member, by any biological criterion, of the human species, although it is only *potentially* an adult actually engaged in the specifically human activities of thinking and willing. But here again, one must distinguish between the passive *potencies* in the fetus (e.g. the capacity of the chemical materials of which it is formed to be combined into various macro-molecules or to be organized into tissues and organs), and its *active* potency as a living thing to develop itself, to differentiate its tissues and organs, to function at various levels, and finally to arrive at full adult functioning as an actually thinking, willing person.

The essential fact is that this active potency by which the zygote is developed into a human person exists not in some external agent (the mother or society) but is inherent in the structure and the genetic code of the zygote itself. From a biological point of view the parent(s) produce the actual zygote, but the zygote transforms itself into the adult organism which is unambiguously a person. Must it not be admitted therefore, that the zygote is actually in a very significant sense a human person, since it is in the process of self-actualization? After all, even the adult person exists as a willing, thinking person only in this process of personal self-development. To be a human person is not to be something absolutely actualized and completed, but to be in a process of actualization. The sleeping person is in the process of resting himself or herself so that he or she will be able to think and will more effectively. The fetal person is in the process of developing the organs necessary for such adult activity.

Of course, the development of certain individual characteristics in the span of total human development is contingent upon circumstances and free choice; e.g. whether this person becomes in adult life a carpenter or a mathematician. But to be human rather than non-human is determined by the presence of the active potentiality to become an adult human which is present with the unique genetic code at conception. There is, however, an important distinction between *remote* and *proximate* potentialities. Thus, for example, in an apple seed, the flowers and future seed are actively potential but only in a remote way. Proximately, the apple seed is in active potency to differentiate into a seedling, and after that into a tree with branches and leaves. So, too, the fetus is in proximate potentiality to develop its anatomical structures, and especially its central nervous system, as necessary preparation to carry out those human activities which will *manifest* his/her personhood.

The epigenetic theory of embryology is precisely the contention that an organism does not develop by a mere unfolding or expansion of already contained structures, but by a stepwise actualization, in which, as each level of organization is actually realized, the next step becomes present in *active potentiality.* Thus the human fetus is only remotely in potentiality for the specifically human functions of rational thought and free will, but is already in the process of developing its central nervous system and the whole anatomical and physiological basis for such rational life. Without this innate active power to develop its own ultimate capacity for personal life, the fetus, no matter how carefully provided for by the human community, would never become an adult member of the community.[33]

At this point the analysis of the beginning of personhood can be summarized as follows:

a. If one asserts that the origin of human personhood is at the moment of conception when a new organic system is present, containing the active potentiality of developing into an adult person under the epigenetic guidance of the information provided by its unique genetic code, this offers a philosophically coherent view based on all available empirical evidence, and one thoroughly cognizant of the dynamic, processive character of living things;

b. If one asserts that human personhood originates after conception, there remains the formidable task of explaining at what point and through what agency this radical change takes place.

We have not yet established that the acceptance of conception as the beginning of personhood necessarily rules out the ethical acceptability of abortion or of non-therapeutic fetal experimentation. It could still be argued that between two persons, one who is well-developed and another who is still at an early stage of the development, the value and rights of the former should be preferred to those of the latter. However, such a discrimination, at least as regards the basic right to live and develop, is contrary to the principle of moral equality of human persons, the argumentation for which is presented in Chapter V, and which has been accepted by the National Commission, as will be shown in Chapter VI.

Delayed Hominization and Personhood. Theories of delayed hominization undertake the "formidable task" mentioned above, namely, to determine and explain at what point and by what process personhood is initiated in the human being *after* conception. Therefore, two of these theories will now be briefly reviewed.

The first of these is an attempt to revive the Aristotelian theory of "mediate animation" (or in current terminology "delayed hominization") which has had great influence in Christian moral theology because of its adoption by St. Thomas Aquinas. Aristotle believed the embryo at first to be only a vegetable organism, which, later, at a point between 40 and 60 days, became radically transformed into a human being with an intellectual soul. Joseph Donceel, S. J., using principles derived from the process philosophy of Teilhard de Chardin and further developed by theologians Karl Rahner and Piet Schoonenberg, has attempted to demonstrate the plausibility of this theory (freed of its obsolete biological data) when placed in an evolutionary context.[34] A detailed and carefully documented study of this theory is presented in Appendix I of this volume. However, a brief resumé of its current status is included here.

If one living species has evolved out of a lower species, why not conceive of the human person as similarly evolving out of several stages of fetal life? Does not this confirm the Aristotelian-Thomistic insistence that a higher form of soul cannot be actually present in matter until that matter has first been prepared for it by a succession of lower forms? In such a conception God, as Author of the whole of nature, is the ultimate cause of the entire evolutionary process which he effects by natural agencies up to the final step, the creation of the human, spiritual person, and this only after the rest of the biological process has been completed. James Diamond, M.D., has supported this position by numerous arguments from embryology which, he believes, indicate a significant threshold at implantation or soon after.[35] Thus, for approximately the first three weeks, according to Diamond, the embryo is non-human. Donceel, however, would place this radical change even later, at the point that the cerebral cortex first appears.

The principal supporting argument for delayed hominization is the fact that before implantation, the human zygote can divide into "identical" twins and perhaps, as some observations with animal zygotes suggest, these twins, in some cases, may recombine into a single viable individual.

From these data it is argued that at this stage, the zygote cannot be a definitively unified organism. How, then, could it be an ensouled person? Where does the second soul originate and what happens to it in the case of recombination? This argument is especially impressive to those who think in dualistic terms of God infusing a soul into a body prepared for it. Here only a brief reply will be given in answer to these difficulties.

First, modern theories of evolution would no longer emphasize the parallel between evolution and embryology, since the old dictum "ontogeny recapitulates phylogeny" is valid only in a very broad sense. Evolution takes place by the natural selection of genetic mutations in a population. Embryological development takes place in an individual organism as an expression of a genetic code intrinsic to the individual and already determined at fertilization. One must not confuse the "evolution of species" with the quite different "epigenetic development."

Second, the plausibility of Aristotle's theory rested on two premises: (1) In a unified substance there must be a proportion of the matter to the form; (2) The matter out of which the fetus is formed has a very much lower level of organization than the highly "tempered" matter which composes the human sense organs on which specifically human functions depend. The first of these premises is a philosophical principle which remains defensible today; but the second has been disproved by modern research. Aristotle supposed that the fetus was formed out of menstrual blood which was non-living but well-digested nutritive material. It is now a scientific fact that the fertilized ovum is a living organism having the same level of organization as any somatic cell in the parental bodies, and containing all the information and active potentiality requisite to develop into an adult human person, as described above.

Third, the various arguments which attempt to show that the pre-implantation zygote is not an individuated human organism fail to explain precisely what occurs at implantation by which it is finally individuated. Certainly, the mother is not the agent of this individuation, since she merely plays the role of host. There seems no doubt that it is the genetic information in the zygote itself that causes it to develop to the twinning point, and which also enables it to implant itself in the uterine wall and to continue developing there in such a way that twinning is no longer possible.

From a strictly biological point of view, the occasional phenomenon of twinning in the development of the human zygote is most plausibly explained as a developmental accident by which some cells become separated from the original zygote and begin to develop into a second, new organism. This process is similar to asexual reproduction in plants or to the "cloning" of a complete animal from the body cells of another. After implantation the zygote is sufficiently differentiated not to be liable to such accidents. The process of recombination seems simply to be the reabsorption of the matter of one of the twins into that of the other. Such developmental accidents are quite intelligible biologically without claiming that the zygote before implantation is a mere collection of cells without organic identity. This supposition offers no explanation of how such a collection of cells follows a definite developmental pathway, or what fuses them at implantation into a single unified individual.

As for the problem of where the second soul originates or where does it go, what difficulty is there in supposing that God, as the Author of nature, creates a soul for the twin when it appears as a distinct organism, just as He did for the first zygote? Or, in the case of recombination, why not suppose that one of the ensouled twins dies and its matter is absorbed by the other, since many zygotes never reach term anyway?

It should be added that those, like Paul Ramsey in recent writings, who connect the origin of personhood with the appearance of the "primary organizer" in the embryo, or who, like Joseph Donceel, associate it with the appearance of the cerebral cortex, fail to take fully into account the epigenetic character of embryological development. For the ultimate "primary organizer" of this entire development is the original nucleus of the fertilized zygote.

While these biological theories of delayed hominization may give comfort to ethicists faced with finding solutions to difficult moral problems involving the abortion issue, they are quite unsatisfying to anyone who, having a clear philosophical understanding of the various uses of the term "human person," also recognizes the epigenetic character of embryological development.

A second type of theory which places the origin of personhood after conception was indicated above in citations from Engelhardt, who has written that, "If the human fetus is more than an 'it,' 'it' surely does not show itself as a person. At most, the fetus is an animal with great promise of becoming more than just an animal."[36] Engelhardt holds that only the adult functioning in self-consciousness and self-determination is unequivocally a person. Why then value the child as human and recognize it as a subject of human rights? He argues that this assignment of value is merely by the community's imputation, although it is not merely arbitrary, since from birth adults begin to interact with the child in an ever-increasingly personal way.[37]

It is necessary to concede in this regard, as has already been done above, that a human being can neither come into existence nor can it develop except in the context of human community. Yet it is also clear that the mother cannot relate *personally* to her newborn unless it is already a *human* person, albeit an infant, not merely in promise, but in actuality. Its "promise" is precisely its own inherent active potentiality to develop into an *adult* person given a suitable biological and social environment.

The imputation theory ignores the priority of personhood to personal interrelations. A personal relation presupposes the existence of two persons, even granting that it is through personal relations that personhood develops to its fullness. The whole moral dilemma of abortion arises precisely because the mother experiences pregnancy as a growth of something alien within herself. Is it alien as a tumor, a diseased part of her body? Rather, she recognizes it as an incipient, independent, healthy organism like herself, which will, therefore, soon make personal demands upon her care. It is precisely the burden of this personal relation and the moral obligations it entails that can make pregnancy so serious a challenge. Any sociological or ethical analysis which glosses over the full complexity of this human situation is entirely inadequate.

Personalist philosophers have balanced their belief in the dynamic process of human growth and development with an equally strong belief in the continuing identity of the person as the ontological basis for that same growth and development. They accept the notion of the person as a complete substance as soon as a unique individual organism of the human species comes into existence. However, by saying "complete" one must not fail also to acknowledge that the fetus may exist in a very undifferentiated way as it begins to grow and develop by its own inner tendency or active potency into a specific kind of living being.

Thus a cautious but well-substantiated answer by a personalist community to the question, Is the human fetus a person? must be a qualified "yes." The fetus is a person-in-process who will not be able to carry on the uniquely human activities of intellection and free choice as a part of a human community, until, with the assistance of that community, it has reached the use of reason through a complex sequence of changes. Yet these changes complete, rather than interrupt its continuous existence as a self-identical being. From conception it exists as a human being with an internal active power of developing into an adult person, and consequently from the beginning it makes a moral demand on the community because it already shares in the life of that community. It is a developing person among developing persons, all of whom are such only because they are giving and receiving members of that community. What the growing fetus gives to the community is indeed a promise, the promise of the community's own future, and that is a very precious contribution.

It should be noted that the above reasoning has vigorously affirmed the beginning of the personhood process at conception. Even the two kinds of delayed hominization theories just outlined would not automatically support the practice of non-therapeutic fetal experimentation before hominization. To whatever degree such theories recognize the continuity of fetal development and the significance of the characteristic "human" applied to the conceptus and pre-hominized fetus, to that degree such theories will discourage its exploitation. A further discussion of this question must now be undertaken: Should the adult community protect the fetus?

Fetal Protection in the Personalist Community

The human community is not an abstract entity on a level over and above human persons. Rather, as was stated, it is the association and interrelation of human persons. Persons are prior to the community in the sense that actual persons are required for its constitution, yet, conversely, community is prior to a particular person, in that he or she is born into an already existing community and can fully realize himself or herself only through participation in the life of that community. This mutual dependence of persons on community and of community on persons shows that they are strict correlatives. One's notion of "community" depends upon the understanding of "person" and vice versa.

Community exists for the development of its members. The relations that form community are not only between persons in their *actuality,* but also in their potentiality. Human community is, accordingly, not primarily a static relationship between persons, but rather a dynamic, changing relationship between individuals whose personal development is not yet complete. Seen from this perspective, communities are just as much "in process" as persons are, since they, too, change in proportion as their members develop or actualize their potentialities for full personhood.

The alternatives to such a dynamic person-centered view of society were seen by the French Thomistic philosopher Jacques Maritain as either an atomistic and mechanistic pattern of bourgeois individualism which eventually destroys the social totality, or a statist or racist totalitarian conception which completely subordinates the person.[38] He saw the common good of a community as their "communion in good living." Included in this, as an essential element, is the "maximum possible development, here and now, of the persons making up the united multitude to the end of forming a people, organized not by force alone but by justice."[39]

The person-centered community, although utopian in its fullest realization, is a direct community of life that binds person to person. The "other" person now acquires the value of an end and purpose rather than the value of a mere means or instrument. Ultimately this is not a community of having but of being. It is not simply a coexistence of individuals each of whom pursues his own happiness along the lines of the "right of privacy" embodied in the *Roe* v. *Wade* Supreme Court decision. The human community does not exist only instrumentally to achieve economic or technological goals; essentially it exists as a normative ideal to make it possible for persons to freely fulfill their personal destiny. Emmanuel Mounier sums up this view of community and persons: "The primary action of the person is to sustain, together with others, a society of persons, the structure, the customs, the sentiments and the institutions of which are shaped by their nature as persons."[40]

Combining this view of the necessary correlation of community and person with the previous conclusion that the human fetus is already a person-in-process from conception produces a clear obligation on the part of the adult community to protect the fetus in its midst. Naturally, this obligation falls first of all upon the parents. Pregnancy, as Albert Outler notes, originates from a social relation between man and woman, not from a mere biological event.[41] Even a rape is a *human* event, although a violently distorted one. The parents, therefore, are the most significant "other persons" for the fetus at that point. Yet a secondary responsibility for the welfare of the conceptus certainly belongs to the community as a whole, but more particularly to its governing group, especially in those instances where the parents do not accept or entirely fulfill their obligations. For, according to the *principle of subsidiarity,* only when there is the failure to meet a responsibility by a lower unit of the community is there a right and an obligation of higher authority to remedy the situation.[42]

With regard to community protection of the fetus, one cannot ignore the present situation in the United States whereby "abortion on demand" is, within certain limits, protected by law. This means that the community has, for all intents and purposes, abdicated protection of the fetus in those cases where the mother herself first abdicated responsibility. Moreover, as noted in Chapter II of this study, the practice of non-therapeutic fetal experimentation as a result of relaxed abortion laws would seem to imply a further step in the progressive degradation of the fetus. For the fetus would thus be not only *rejected* by the mother but *subjected* to the desire of the community at large for the sake of the advance in medical technology. Put in other terms, the mother's personal choice for an abortion becomes a matter of public exploitation, when the community chooses to *use* this fetus and others of its class for the possible presumed benefit of future fetuses.

The irony of such a situation can be seen by citing the statement in the 1972 Supreme Court decision against capital punishment: "In comparison to all other punishments today, then, the deliberate extinction of human life by the State is uniquely degrading to human dignity."[43] Could it not also be argued that the funding of non-therapeutic fetal experimentation by the State (as government) would be even more drastically "degrading to human dignity?" While charges of a consequent "brutalization," either of the medical profession or of society at large, are difficult to prove in advance of actual experience, the "wedge" argument therein implied does not lack weight. That is, there exists already in society today considerable fear of patient exploitation by those medical technologists and doctors who have abandoned the intimacy and trust of the traditional patient/physician relationship. What then would be the long range effects on the public, given governmental approval for (unrestricted, nontherapeutic) fetal experimentation? The State, in any case, needs to exercise great caution here, since one of its principal roles in society has always been to safeguard the community as a whole from the excesses of its individual members, even when they were presumably acting in the public interest.

In concluding this discussion of the dynamics of person, community, and the position of the fetus in the community of persons, some general observations can be made about the perspective of a person-centered community toward the fetus which will be useful in Chapter VI.

The laudable contemporary efforts to improve the quality of human life must not lead to a sliding scale of human value which is directly proportioned to the utility or function of persons within the community. Lord Dawson, in speaking to the British Parliament, frankly described this sliding scale: "This is a courageous age, but it has a different sense of values from the ages which have gone before. It looks upon life more from the point of view of quality than of quantity. It places less value on life when its usefulness has come to an end."[44] No authentically person-centered community, however, can measure out the worth of its members, especially its weakest ones, on a scale of health, intelligence, or any similar "quality of life" index. Any such effort reduces the basis of personhood of the community members to the sole criterion of utility, much as workers in a factory are measured by productive output.

Linked with the unfortunate trend to equate *value* of life with *quality* of life in the present situation is the trend to value the fetus affirmatively or negatively, depending on whether or not it is "wanted" by its progenitors. The implication of this false value-norm is that individual persons are assigned their ultimate value by other individual persons in their surroundings. Obviously individual persons do establish their own value-relationships with one another. But personhood brings with it a more profound value which cannot be given or taken away by other persons. Jean Moroux, the French philosopher, explained this value in philosophical terms: "A thing that exists for itself is one that has a meaning and a value of its own, which is ordered to itself, which is an end, with an absolute, definitive and unique character in the universe."[46] This does not mean, of course, that human life has an absolute value; communities have traditionally defended themselves against unjust aggression even at the cost of life to some of their members. But the implication of Moroux's comments is that *human persons possess an intrinsic and existential value regardless of relative value that might be attributed to them by other members of the community.* Not only do individuals have certain duties toward the community, but the community itself must assume a definite stance of responsibility toward the individual. The community, in other words, is obligated to protect each person's right to fulfill his or her destiny. As Thomas P. Neill wrote at the end of World War II, "man's only right, in the last analysis, is the right to be a man, to live as a human person."[47] When, therefore, the basic right to life of one whole class of persons within the community is notably jeopardized, then the community as a whole is endangered. With the *Roe v. Wade* decision of the Supreme Court in January, 1973, the basic right to life of the human fetus has been seriously called into question.

In brief, the clear and unequivocal answer to the question, Should the adult community protect the fetus as likewise a person? is, without a doubt, "yes." A person-centered community which treats its members as ends and subjects, not merely as means and objects, will also consider fetuses as subjects and ends even though they are just in the initial stages of personhood. Whatever practical guidelines are developed for fetal experimentation must not lose sight of this personalist perspective.

Summary

A personalistic or person-centered community is one composed of human individuals who participate in a shared life as freely developing and mutually interacting members. An analysis of those beings who are indubitably persons—e.g., awake, alert, normal human adults—reveals that they are unique individuals with the power of self-determination who nonetheless require interaction with other humans for the unfolding, expression and completion of that unreplicable personhood; hence the absolute need for human community.

From this perspective, is the human fetus a person *in any sense*? The specific biological uniqueness of the fetus is determined at its earliest stages when the zygote is constituted by the fusion of the human parental egg and sperm to form the zygote with the full genetic program for human development. The fetus' power of self-determination is present as an *active* capacity whose presence is increasingly manifest as it proceeds without significant discontinuities through various developmental stages to mature adulthood (unless impeded by accident, disease or defect). There is no evidence of a radical change occurring *after* conception when the actual potency of human self-development is granted to it by some external power. Consequently, the fetus can be properly denominated a person, even if its *manifestations* are still largely potential.

Even if the various philosophical theories of delayed hominization are given some credit (and they are not very plausible) the fetus from conception must be granted human value as a human being in the process of becoming a functioning person by an inherent natural tendency. From a personalist point of view this leads to the conclusion that the community must acknowledge the ethical demand made by the existence of the fetus as a person-in-process from conception and must afford it the protection and opportunity for development which are the basic rights of every person. To do less would be to accept as a principle that the community can deny these rights to human beings on grounds other than their own rejection of that community.

Because the human community is itself in process, developing in proportion as its individual members develop their potentialities for full personhood, it has a necessary concern for the well-being of all those who have the active potentiality for such development. Such concern should extend to the protection of fetuses—*those members, who, while they appear to be the most helpless and least useful, are yet the ones on whom the future of the community depends.*

CHAPTER III Footnotes

1. Pannenberg, Wolfhart, *What Is Man?*, Philadelphia: Fortress Press, 1970, p. 83.
2. *Ibid.*

3. *A Catholic-Humanist Dialogue,* Kurtz, Paul and Dondeyne, Albert, editors, Buffalo: Prometheus Books, 1972, p. 3.
4. *Ibid.*
5. Documents of Vatican II, Abbott, Walter M., SJ, editor, New York: Guild Press, 1966, p. 224.
6. See Di Ianni, Albert R., "Is the Fetus a Person?" *American Ecclesiastical Review* 168(5):309-326, May, 1975.
7. *In Cancer Ward,* New York: Farrar, Strauss, and Geroux, Inc., 1968, Bantam Books, p. 428.
8. Rahner, Karl, SJ, *Theological Investigations,* Vol. II, Baltimore: Helicon Press, Third Printing, 1966, p. 239.
9. "The two kinds of twins just referred to (dizygotic and monozygotic twins) are usually called 'fraternal' and 'identical'. Identical, however, is too strong an adjective. No two individuals, not even the most similar of twins, are alike in every detail (i.e., 'identical')." Moody, Paul A., *Genetics of Man,* New York: W. W. Norton & Co., Inc., 1967, p. 288.
10. See Premack, A. J. and Premack, David, "Teaching Language to an Ape", *Scientific American* 227(4):92-100, October, 1972.
11. See Walgrave, John, *Person and Society*, Pittsburgh: Duquesne University Press, 1965, pp. 97-101.
12. D'Arcy, Martin C., *The Mind and the Heart of Love,* London, 1945, p. 321.
13. Marcel, Gabriel, *The Mystery of Being,* Vol. II, Chicago: Henry Regnery Co., Gateway Edition, 1960, p. 69.
14. *Ibid.*, p. 208.
15. Boethius, *Contra Eutychen,* III, 4.
16. See *Summa Theologica,* P. III, Q. 16. 12, ad 2.
17. Kurtz, Paul and Wilson, Edwin H., "Humanist Manifesto II", *Current,* November, 1973, pp. 28-36; see pp. 33-34.
18. Dupré, Louis, "Philosophical Considerations" in *Beginnings of Personhood,* McCarthy, Donald, editor, Houston, Texas: The Institute of Religion and Human Development, 1973, p. 22.
19. Mahoney, Maurice J. and Associates, Report to the National Commission for the Protection of Human Subjects, March 14, 1975, p. 1. This definition was borrowed from the working papers of the British advisory committee chaired by Sir John Peel.
20. *Federal Register,* 40(154):33531, August 8, 1975
21. Liley, A. W., "The Foetus as Personality", *Australia and New Zealand Journal of Psychiatry* 6:99-105, 1972. Note that this quotation need not impute consciousness or moral freedom on the part of the human fetus.
22. For a discussion of some attempts to discover such crises of radical change in embryological development, see Appendix I.
23. "The Beginnings of Personhood: Theological Considerations", *Perkins Journal of Theology* 27(1):31, Fall, 1973.
24. "Ethical-Theological Aspects of Direct Abortion" in *Theological Studies* 31:128, 1970.
25. "The Morality of Abortion" in *Life or Death: Ethics and Options*, Labby, Daniel, editor, Seattle: University of Washington Press, 1968, p. 69.
26. Mounier, E., *Personalism,* Notre Dame, Ind.: Notre Dame University Press, 1975, p. 11.
27. *Op. cit.,* p. 23.
28. For an account of these modern concepts see von Bertalanffy, Ludwig, *General System Theory,* New York: George Braziller, 1968.
29. Engelhardt, H. Tristram, Jr., "Viability, Abortion, and the Difference between a Fetus and an Infant", *American Journal of Obstetrics and Gynecology* 116:429-434, June, 1973, p. 430.
30. Engelhardt, H. Tristram, Jr., "The Beginnings of Personhood: Philosophical Considerations", *Perkins Journal of Theology* 27:20-27, Fall, 1973, p. 23. Engelhardt is correct in saying that the term "person" unambiguously designates a self-conscious, self-determining, free agent and that it cannot be properly extended to entities such as the

fetus, the child, the senile without warranted criteria for this extension if the term is to be philosophically useful. However, it is absurd to deny that a sleeping adult is not a person; consequently *some* extension of the term to include entities which are "potentially" self-conscious, determining, free agents is clearly necessary. The issue, therefore, becomes the various ways in which persons can exist "potentially". In some senses of potential existence a potential person cannot reasonably be said to have value or rights, e.g., a merely *possible* person, such as "protended grandchildren," "future generations." On the other hand, the sleeping adult certainly has both value and rights. It is essential, therefore, to distinguish the various senses of potentiality and actuality. Certainly many philosophers would think that the fetus is a "who" precisely because it has the intrinsic capacity of self-development by which it will become a person, just as the sleeping adult has the capacity to wake up and begin to think again.

31. *The Ethics of Sex,* New York, 1964, p. 227.
32. *Op. cit.*, p. 20.
33. For a more extensive treatment of this entire subject, see Wade, Francis C., "Potentiality in the Abortion Discussion", *Review of Metaphysics* 22:239-55, 1975.
34. See Donceel, Joseph F., SJ, "Immediate Animation and Delayed Hominization", *Theological Studies* 31:76-105, 1970. Joseph Mangan, SJ, responds to this theory in "The Wonder of Myself: Ethical-in-Theological Aspects of Direct Abortion", *Theological Studies* 31:125-148, 1970, especially pp. 126-134. See Appendix I for detailed analysis of the theory of delayed hominization.
35. Diamond, James J., M.D., "Abortion, Animation, Hominization", *Theological Studies* 36:305-324, 1975.
36. Engelhardt, H. Tristram, Jr., "The Ontology of Abortion", *Ethics*, LXXXIV, 1973—74, P. 220.
37. *Ibid.*, pp. 230-32.
38. See Maritain, J., *The Person and the Common Good*, Notre Dame, Ind.: University of Notre Dame Press, 1972, p. 101.
39. Op. cit., pp. 51, 53-54.
40. *Op. cit.*, p. 21.
41. *Op. cit.*, p. 28.
42. The principle of subsidiarity is discussed more fully by John H. Walgrave in his *Person and Society* (Pittsburgh: Duquesne University Press, pp. 155-163.) As Walgrave observes, Pius XI, in his encyclical *Quadragesimo Anno,* strongly emphasized this principle:

    It is indeed true, as history clearly proves, that owing to the change in social conditions, much that was formerly done by small bodies can nowadays be accomplished only by large corporations. Nonetheless, just as it is wrong to withdraw from the individual and commit to the community at large what private enterprise and industry can accomplish, so, too, it is an injustice, a grave evil and a disturbance of right order for a larger and higher organization to arrogate to itself functions which can be performed efficiently by smaller and lower bodies. This is a fundamental principle of social philosophy, unshaken and unchangeable, and it retains its full truth today. Of its very nature, the true aim of all social activity should be to help individual members of the social body, but never to destroy or absorb them.
43. Furman v. Georgia, 408 U.S. 283; 33 L. Ed. 2d, 346, 378 (1972).
44. Quoted by Ayd, Frank, "Voluntary Euthanasia: The Right to be Killed", *Medical-Moral Newsletter,* January and February, 1970, p. 17.
45. For an excellent discussion of the philosophical background of this position, see Di Ianni, Albert R., "Is the Fetus a Person?", *American Ecclesiastical Review* 168:309-326, 1974, especially pp. 315-16.
46. Mouroux, Jean, *The Meaning of Man,* New York: Doubleday and Co., Image Books, 1961, p. 116.
47. *Weapons for Peace,* Milwaukee: Bruce, 1945, p. 155.

4

The Personal God/Man Relationship and the Fetus in the Christian Community

From the perspective of both the civic community and the personalist community, human values transcend physical nature and empirical measurement because the human person is an end in himself and cannot be reduced to a being of secondary, instrumental value. A genuine humanism welcomes the advance of technology, but it must not succumb to that "technological spirit" described by Pius XII as one which "only recognizes and reckons as real what can be expressed in mathematical formulae and utilitarian calculations."[1]

Anyone who recognizes this transcendent, universal and ultimately mysterious dignity of every human person is forced to cross a value threshold. Personalist thinkers like Albert Camus and Victor Frankl made this step for non-religious reasons. Christian believers do so for religious reasons, but reasons that are completely consistent with the human experiences shared by believers and nonbelievers alike. Therefore the faith-vision of Christian theology seeks to synthesize all the insights concerning the civil rights of members of a civilized society and the dynamic correlation of persons-in-community already discussed in Chapters II and III.

Going further, Christian theology insists that the mystery of human personhood can be understood more profoundly only by realizing that God Himself is personal—supremely personal as the Trinitarian community of divine Persons, and visibly personal in the human presence of Jesus Christ. The supremely personal God is the origin, conserving power, and ultimate fulfillment of each unique created person. Only God can create a person and endow that person with eternal life.[2] Only God's life-giving grace can touch a person at the deepest level of personal existence—the level of freedom—where nature and grace dynamically meet to fully actualize the unique personhood of each individual. This growth of the created person will be consummated only in an intimate relation with God and neighbor in the everlasting community which is the Kingdom of God.

This strictly theological understanding of the dignity of the person will be discussed briefly under four headings: (1) the Biblical teaching on the beginning of personhood and nature of the human person; (2) an historical survey of Catholic theology on the beginnings of personhood; (3) Protestant theology from Luther to the present on the beginning of personhood; (4) Protestant-Catholic divergences and rapprochement.

Biblical Teaching on the Beginnings of Personhood

Contemporary theology does not look to the Bible for "proof-texts" to settle modern problems. Its method is to study fundamental themes which developed historically in the Old and New Testament writings, and then to try to understand the implications of these insights to the problems of human life. There is no point, therefore, in searching the Bible for concrete and clearly defined answers to the problems of embryology, or for a solution to ethical dilemmas about fetal experimentation. Rather the Bible offers an understanding of the religious meaning of human life from the creative act by which God brings each person into being to the hour of death and final judgment.

For the present purpose in this section, it is sufficient to deal briefly with three questions: (a) What is the Creator's personal relation to the individual persons He creates? (b) When does this personal relation begin? (c) What is the specifically New Testament understanding of this relation?

The Creator's Personal Relationship to Each Human Being

The I-Thou Relationship: Pius XII reaffirmed the traditional teaching "that [human] souls are immediately created by God."[3] This implies that the human parents cooperate in the production of the human person by producing the body, and in this respect are instruments of God through whom He acts creatively but *mediately,* but it is only God Himself acting *immediately* who can give spiritual existence and hence personhood to the whole human individual.[4] Thus Catholic tradition affirms that God stands in a much more intimate and immediate relation to each human person than to the plants and animals whom He produces *mediately* through natural causes.

Is this traditional affirmation based on Scriptural teaching?[5] In the Yahwist account in *Genesis 2* according to current exegesis, the author wishes to teach that God, in creating Adam, at once entered into an intimate I-Thou relation with this archetypal human person.[6] Yahweh God forms the animals "out of the ground" (v. 19), and He forms Adam in the same way, but in his case God also "blew into his nostrils the breath of life, and so man became a living being" (v. 7). Thus man lives by the very life-breath of God Himself. This intimate and personal relation between the personal God and the human person is further indicated (v. 17 ff.) by the fact that God speaks to man and gives him the right to name the animals, that is, to share in God's own sovereignty over His creation. Furthermore, by His commandment (v. 15 ff.), God makes man morally responsible as a free being for stewardship over creation.

Yet this immediate relation of God and Adam is not to be understood in a merely individualistic sense. "The Lord God said: 'It is not good for the man to be alone. I will make a suitable partner for him.'" (v. 18) No partner proves suitable except a woman like man himself. Thus a person's humanity is not complete except in relation to another human being, and indeed to the community formed by their offspring, as is made plain in the account in *Genesis* 1, v. 27 f.

Nor can it be supposed that this immediate relation to God was true only of the first human persons. Eve, according to the Yahwist author, on bearing her first child, Cain, cries out, "I have produced a man with the help of the Lord."(4:1) Thus, in the Biblical view of the first chapters of *Genesis,* God is the creator of each human person in an immediate way that establishes that person in an I-Thou relation with God, and at the same time, in relation to the other members of the human community, which is God's people.

The Significance of Personal Names: This basic Biblical theme is brought out in another way throughout the Scriptures by the fact that God gives personal *names* to certain men and women whom He called into existence to perform a unique mission in *His* name. At all times, to call a person by his or her proper name is somehow to establish a personal and even intimate relation. When we do so we speak not merely to an acquaintance, or an official, or a member of a group or a class, but precisely to this *unique* person, whom we know and who knows us directly and immediately in our personhood. This is why, in the story of *Exodus,* it is essential that God reveal His true name to Moses, and that God also calls Moses by *his* name. "The Lord said to Moses: 'This request, too, which you have just made, I will carry out, because you have found favor with me and you are my intimate friend'" [literally: "I know you by name"] (33:17).

God gives or changes the names of the patriarchs to indicate their election as progenitors of the Chosen People. Thus He says to Abram, "'No longer shall you be called Abram; your name shall be Abraham, for I am making you the father of a host of nations'. . . . As for your wife Sarai, do not call her Sarai; her name shall be Sarah. I will bless her, and I will give you a son by her.'" (Genesis 17:5, 15f). Again, "God replied: 'Nevertheless, your wife Sarah is to bear a son, and you shall call him Isaac. I will maintain my covenant with him as an everlasting pact, to be his God and the God of his descendants after him.'"(Genesis 17:19)

> But Jacob said, "I will not let you go until you bless me." "What is your name?" the man asked. He answered, "Jacob." Then the man said, "You shall no longer be spoken of as Jacob, but as Israel, because you have contended with divine and human beings and have prevailed." Jacob then asked him, "Do tell me your name, please." He answered, "Why should you want to know my name?" With that, he bade him farewell. Jacob named the place Peniel (probably 'the face of God'), 'because I have seen God face to face' he said, 'yet my life has been spared.' (32:27b-31).

Thus the name of God and the name of man expresses the covenantal relation, the promise of God, the special gifts of power and knowledge which God grants a human to carry out a mission in His name.

Nor is this naming only for a few special persons. It applies to God's people as a whole and to each member, as the prophets indicate. Thus, in *Isaiah* 62:4, God says to Jerusalem, "No more shall men call you 'Forsaken,' or your land 'Desolate,' but you shall be called 'My Delight,' and your land 'Espoused.'" And in 44:5 the prophet says, "one shall say, 'I am the Lord's,' another shall be named after Jacob, and this one shall write on his hand, 'The Lord's' and Israel shall be his surname." This same idea is found in the many *theophoric* names in the Bible which contain as one element some form of the name of God, "El," "Yah," or "Adonai." "The content of theophoric propositional names is that the divinity: 1) has given, created/made, or added the child named; 2) has granted, helped, saved, and has mercy, spared, restored justice, and cured, or that it may do so."[7] In Hebrew names a second element usually refers to the parents, so that the whole name expresses the mutual relation of God, the child, and the community (the parents).

It is not strange, therefore, that in the New Testament Luke emphasizes that the vocation of John the Baptizer was heralded by the angel Gabriel: "Your prayer has been heard. Your wife Elizabeth shall bear a son whom you shall name John" (*Luke* 1:13b). The same angel tells Mary of her Son's name and vocation: "You have found favor with God. You shall conceive and bear a son and give him the name Jesus" (1:30-31). This is the culminating example, but Jesus continues the principle by giving a new name, "Peter," to His disciple Simon-bar-Jona, to indicate that he is to be chief of the band (*Mark* 3:17; *Matthew* 16:18) and to His other two favorites, James and John, the sons of Zebedee, whom He called, "The Sons of Thunder" (*Mark* 3:17).

This practice was continued in the early Church by the custom of the baptismal name, in place of the name given at circumcision (*Luke* 2:21), as marking Christian regeneration and the call to witness to the Gospel even at the price of martyrdom. "To the victor I will give the hidden manna; I will give him a white stone upon which is inscribed a new name, to be known only by him who receives it" (*Revelations* 2:17). "I will make the victor a pillar in the temple of my God and he shall never leave it. I will inscribe on him the name of my God and the name of the city of my God, the new Jerusalem which he will send down from heaven, and my own name which is new" (Revelation 3:12). In this last text, note that the "new name" is at once the name of God, of Jesus, and of the "new Jerusalem," i.e., the community of the elect, because it indicates the fulfillment of the covenant relation, the perfect communication of the Divine Life to all.

Thus the Biblical indication that God gives names to His people implies His direct and immediate concern for them as individuals. The implication that God knows each of His persons substantiates the Biblical teaching of *Genesis* about His direct involvement in the creation of every person.

The Temporal Beginning of the Personal Relationship

It seems obvious from the above discussion that the Bible teaches that the I-Thou relationship of God to each human person in creation and re-creation (redemption) is both intimately personal and also communitarian. But when does this relation begin? It is hardly to be expected that the Bible would be concerned with embryological details, yet a study of the texts does show a definite orientation in Biblical thought:

> Before I formed you in the womb I Knew you, before you were born I dedicated you, a prophet of the nations I appointed you. (*Jeremiah* 1:5)

Similarly in the great *Psalm* 22, (which Jesus recited on the Cross according to *Mark* 15:34), the Psalmist says:

> You have been my guide since I was first formed,
> [Or more literally: Yet you drew me out of the womb]
> my security at my mother's breast.
> To you I was committed at birth,
> From my mother's womb you are my God.

This is closely connected with the theme of vocation and naming already discussed. Thus the prophet Isaiah (or, more likely, the Deutero-Isaiah) says,"The Lord called me from my birth, from my mother's womb he gave me my name" (49:1). He also pictures God calling Cyrus, as a type of the Messiah:

> Thus says the Lord, your redeemer, who formed you from the womb (44:24 a). . . . That you may know that I am the Lord, the God of Israel, who calls you by your name. For the sake of Jacob, my servant, of Israel my chosen one, I have called you by our name, giving you a title, though you knew me not. (45:3-4)

Thus the Biblical writers see God as the author of the entire process by which a human person comes into existence. He wills that this unique person come into existence in relation to Him from the beginning, so that what God wills is *this* person, with a special destiny in relation to Him. The notion that the parents produce a body into which God then infuses a soul does not do justice to this Biblical conception. Again *Psalm* 139 says:

> Truly you have formed my inmost being [literally: my kidneys]:
> you knit me in my mother's womb.
> I give you thanks that I am fearfully, wonderfully made;
> wonderful are your works.
> My soul also you knew full well;
> nor was my frame unknown to you
> when I was made in secret,
> when I was fashioned in the depths of the earth.
> Your eyes have seen my actions [*in Hebrew:* My embryo];
> in your book they are all written;
> my days are limited before one of them existed (13-16).

In this vivid passage, "depths of the earth" means "in the womb." The term "kidneys" is equivalent to "heart," not merely in the physical sense, but in the sense of "inmost being." The phrase "my soul" refers to the *nepes* which means "the whole living man in his neediness."[8] The last three lines present some textual problems, but the Massoretic text refers to the "embryo," or as Wolff translates, "primal form."

In a similar passage, *Job* says:

> Your hands have formed me and fashioned me;
> will you then turn and destroy me?
> Oh, remember that you fashioned me from clay!
> Will you then bring me down to dust again?
> Did you not pour me out as milk,
> and thicken me like cheese?
> With skin and flesh you clothed me,
> with bones and sinews knit me together.
> Grace and favor you granted me,
> and your providence has preserved my spirit. (10:8-12).

In *2 Maccabees* the heroic mother of seven sons recalls this doctrine as a motive for a martyr's faith in the resurrection, when she says to her youngest son:

> I do not know how you came into existence in my womb;
> it was not I who gave you the breath of life, nor was
> it I who set in order the elements of which each of you is
> composed. Therefore, since it is the Creator of the universe
> who shapes each man's beginning, as he brings
> about the origin of everything, he, in his mercy, will

give you back both breath and life, because you now
disregard yourselves for the sake of his law
(7:22-23).

This language leaves no doubt that the Biblical writers see God as forming the whole being of the individual person, not merely anatomically, but in his or her inmost being as a person from the very beginning of the reproductive process and it even connects this with the ultimate resurrection to eternal life.

This same outlook under a different aspect is found again in the famous verse of *Psalm* 51:5:

Indeed, in guilt was I born,
and in sin my mother conceived me . . .

This verse is not saying that the sexual act is sinful, a notion foreign to the Old Testament, but is teaching that the human person comes into existence in an earthly world of physical fragility and liability to disease, death, ritual uncleanness, and moral fallibility.[9] This means that the human person stands under the judgment of God, not only from birth, but from *conception* (emphasized by the climactic parallelism of these verses). The term for "conception" here refers to the animal heat of physical intercourse, and thus emphasizes the early emergence of the new human being.

Thus it seems clear that, according to the Old Testament view, the I-Thou relation of each unique human being with God begins from the very inception of the creative process by which the human organism comes into existence. Despite this belief, Rabbinic tradition was able to permit abortion according to a legal casuistry based on a single text from *Exodus.*[10] This legal compromise could not override the profound doctrine on God's creative will for man, any more than the legal provisions for divorce could cancel out the teaching of *Genesis* on God's will for the relation of man and woman, as Jesus later emphasized (*Mark* 10:2-9). The development of religious and ethical understanding in the Old Testament, culminating in the New Testament, tends always to overcome such compromise in favor of a higher and deeper understanding.

The New Testament View of This Relationship

The Central Role of the Doctrine of the Incarnation: Nothing has more deeply influenced the specifically Christian understanding of the beginnings of personhood than the doctrine of the Incarnation, the central event of human history in which "the Word was made flesh," the Son of God became Jesus of Nazareth. However, this central Biblical theme is also bound up with other themes very prominent in Christian tradition, but which today are relegated by many theologians, both Protestant and Catholic, to the periphery of Christian teaching. To the contemporary mind, these themes, such as the infancy narratives of Matthew and Luke, the doctrine of the "virgin birth" of Jesus, the Catholic doctrine of the Immaculate Conception of Mary herself, and the various theologies of infant baptism and original sin, seem so entangled with mythological or legendary elements as to become almost meaningless.

Recent theological work, however, is beginning to face these questions honestly, and to seek out the deeper theological significance of the infancy narratives. Although the earliest level of the New Testament writings, such as the epistles of St. Paul and the Gospel according to St. Mark, put little emphasis on this aspect of Christology, the interest in the earthly origins of Jesus manifested by the Gospels of St. Luke and St. Matthew show that Christians very early began to meditate on such themes and their practical spiritual consequences for Christian self-understanding.

The I-Thou relation of the Israelite to God which the Yahwist pondered was soon seen by Christians to be their own relation, as individual persons and as a community of persons, to the Father through the Spirit in the Son, Jesus Christ, true God and true human. Christians through baptism enter into the Triune Community, which is the One God, through incorporation into the Incarnate Word. Furthermore, this entrance of human persons into divine communion is achieved *historically* through unique events in which every Christian participates. Consequently, the biographies of the patriarchs, the prophets, of John the Baptizer, of Mary, of Jesus and the individual biographies of Christians from the moment of entrance into existence until passage through death to resurrection are theologically significant. Christian understanding of human life cannot deal merely with abstract ideals of the "mature person," but must arise from a meditation on the total process by which they become actualized persons in a community—a "kingdom be-come" in eschatological fulfillment.

The Incarnation and the Personhood of Christ: Thus it no longer appears strange that, while the early preaching of St. Paul concentrated so entirely on the mystery of the Cross and Resurrection, by the time St. Luke composed his Gospel, he was concerned that the story of Jesus be completed by pondering theologically and synthesizing the traditions of how Jesus came to be, and how His Church became His continuing presence in the world.[11] It is Luke who gave to Christian thought its basic theology of the Incarnation as an event in salvation history, and thus provided a paradigm for understanding the initiation of human personhood. He does so by placing the Annunciation to Mary in the context of the Old Testament themes already studied.[12] Furthermore, in the scene of the Visitation of the pregnant Mary to the pregnant Elizabeth (*Luke* 1:39-55), Elizabeth is filled with the spirit of prophecy through the future prophet in her womb, and she proclaims the presence of the Lord in Mary's womb. Hence the culminating moment of all history, the Incarnation of the Son of God, is recognized by the revealing spirit as already begun in Mary, who thus became the new Temple of God, in which the Shekinah or Divine Presence is already manifest.[13]

Thus Jesus in His Divine Personhood is present as truly human from the very time of His conception. Yet, for Luke, this unique fact is also realized in an analogical way in the merely human John the Baptizer. Thus, it is the Christian conviction that *every* human being, from the moment that the divine creative action effects the immediate creation of that unique individual, is in a personal relation to God. The history of salvation includes all human beings as members of a single community in which Jesus is head and pattern of the whole.

Another important approach to the concern for the unborn would be to consider the fact that the Gospel is for the poor and the oppressed first of all. As Jacques Dupont and others have recently shown in their study of the concept of the Kingdom of God and of the Beatitudes, the texts relating to the "little ones" and the "little child" (who is the model of all those who enter the Kingdom) teach that the basic attitude of Jesus, and therefore of all who take discipleship seriously, is "care for the helpless and dispossessed." In the present context, that would include concern also for the rights of the unborn.

In summarizing this review of Biblical teaching about the beginnings of personhood it must be admitted that the Scriptures do not speak specifically about personhood, beginning at conception. However, the Scriptures do teach, not in isolated proof texts, but in a profound, thematic manner, intimately related to the most fundamental doctrines of Christian faith, that God's role in the Creation and Redemption of each unique human being begins before birth, indeed from the very moment that such an individual begins to be. This Biblical valuation of the human being lays on the human community a very grave obligation to receive this divine gift of human life and to protect and cherish it.

Historical Survey of Catholic Theology on the Beginnings of Personhood

The early Christian community, growing in an environment whose values were frequently in conflict with their own, had to face a number of theoretical and practical problems, among which were the common practices of contraception and abortion. Over the centuries to the very present, those problems have remained and have required periodic review. And it is these issues, particularly that of abortion, which in the past have made the question of the beginning of personhood of more than theoretical interest. Today, the practice of fetal experimentation and the possiblities of genetic manipulation have given added impetus to this concern about the genesis of personhood.

An accurate and illuminating account of the history of Catholic teaching and practice on the origin of personhood can be found in the essay of John T. Noonan Jr., the American historian and law professor, "An Almost Absolute Value in History"; other recent studies essentially confirm his account, with some differences in interpretation.[14] Here it will suffice to summarize this research by pointing out that there have been three several stages of development in Catholic thinking on this subject.

Patristic Period to Pius IX

First, in the patristic period of the *Church,* there is ample evidence, both in sermons and church legislation, that abortion and infanticide alike were viewed as grave sins for which someone could be justly excluded from membership in the Christian community. Thus, what is probably the earliest extra-Biblical manual of Christian ethical standards, the *Didache,* commands: "Thou shalt not procure abortion, nor commit infanticide."[15] Tertullian (c. 160-c. 220) eloquently expressed this general point of view:

> For us (Christians), indeed, just as homicide is forbidden, so it is not lawful to destroy what is conceived in the womb while the blood is still being formed into a man. To prevent being born is to accelerate homicide, nor does it make a difference whether you snatch away a soul which is born or destroy one being born. He who is man-to-be is man, as all fruit is now in the seed.[16]

At this state, therefore, the Christian respect for human life at every stage of development was quite unambiguous. However, the writers of this period did not deal explicitly either with the distinction between contraception and abortion, or the precise time of the "infusion of the human soul."

Second, in the medieval period this tradition was maintained, but the canon lawyers and scholastic theologians, such as Thomas Aquinas, became concerned with the technical problem of the classification of the sin of abortion in view of confessional judgment and canonical penalties. Is abortion a species of homicide, or a different type of sin, something intermediate between illicit contraception and infanticide? In attempting to solve such questions they made use of two distinctions which seemed to them plausible. From Jewish tradition reflected in the Greek translation of *Exodus* 21:22, they accepted the distinction in value between a "formed" and an "unformed" fetus. From Aristotelian embryology, they accepted the distinction among a vegetative, animal and human stage of animation of the fetus, so that at least before the fortieth day of pregnancy the fetus was not informed by a truly human soul. Thus they concluded that abortion at this early stage before human ensoulment was not technically homicide, but that it was still a very grave sin against nature, more serious than contraception.

Third, in the Renaissance and post-Tridentine period, theologians, concerned with the development of a practical casuistic moral theology, gave explicit attention to conflict situations in which the rights of mother and child have to be balanced, or where doubts arise about the duty to baptize the fetus. At first, out of respect to the medieval authorities who had accepted the Aristotelian theory, many theologians, including even the great St. Alphonsus Ligouri, taught that there is some ethical probability to the view that therapeutic abortions may be permitted in some difficult cases. Some laxists even taught that it might be justified to save the reputation of the mother (equivalent to modern "psychiatric reasons"). Nevertheless, the Holy See continued to oppose abortion and impose sanctions against it, while not decisively repudiating the more liberal theological opinions.[17]

Pius IX to Paul VI

The development of scientic embryology, however, gradually destroyed the plausibility of the Aristotelian theory on which these more liberal opinions rested. Joseph Donceel, S. J., and others have argued that this change of opinion was based more on the influence of Cartesian dualism and preformist theories of embryology than on empirical data.[18] However, this seems unlikely since the first influential attack against the Aristotelian view was made by Paolo Zacchis, in 1621, some 16 years before Descartes had published his first philosophical work. Further, as shown in Appendix I below, the empirical evidence against Aristotle soon became very impressive and has continued to increase to the present time. The formal rejection of delayed ensoulment as a general teaching of the Church came in 1869, when Pius IX, in the constitution *Apostolicae Sedis,* dropped the reference to "ensouled fetus" in the excommunication for abortion so that the excommunication now applies to abortion of any embryo or fetus of human parentage.

Beginning in 1884, the Holy Office began explicitly to exclude *in practice* the liberal casuistic theories, without, however, condemning the *theory* of delayed hominization in itself. In the recent *Declaration of Abortion,* of the Sacred Congregation for the Doctrine of the Faith, November 18, 1974, an interesting note explains this as follows:

> This declaration expressly leaves aside the question of the moment when the spiritual soul is infused. There is not a unanimous tradition on this point and authors are as yet in disagreement. For some it dates from the first instant, for others it could not at least precede nidation. It is not within the competence of science to decide between these views, because the existence of an immortal soul is not a question in its field. It is a philosophical problem from which our moral affirmation remains independent for two reasons: (1) supposed a belated animation, there is still nothing less than a *human* life preparing for and calling for a soul in which the nature received from parents is completed; (2) on the other hand it suffices that this presence of the soul be probable (and one can never prove the contrary) in order that the taking of life involves accepting the risk of killing a man, not only waiting for, but already in possession of his soul.[19]

Noonan's interpretation of this whole third period of development seems well-grounded when he writes:

> This development represented a substantial return to the patristic

prohibition without the glosses and exceptions written in by casuistry, but it was not a naive invocation of the past; it was a conscious rejection of some solutions which had once been appealing. Hence, it was a development—a testing of principles by human experience in the light of the Gospel and reformulation of doctrine after this testing. Like other developed Christian teaching on slavery, on the rights of labor, on war, it embodied a sensitivity to certain values affirmed in the Gospel but not made effective in Roman, medieval, or post-Reformation culture.[20]

The adoption of this stricter view by the Popes from the time of Pius IX is clear in all the more recent documents of the Holy See, beginning with Pius XII, who had special interest in medical-moral problems. Thus in his 1951 address to midwives, he said, "Once man has fulfilled his part and set in motion the marvelous evolution of life, it is his duty to respect religiously its progress . . ."[21] He goes on to reject all doubts about the human personhood of the fetus, "Now even the unborn child is 'man' *to the same degree* and by the same title as the mother" (italics added).

That same year, in another address, Pius XII referred to the inviolability of innocent human life:

> Innocent life, in whatsoever condition it is found, is withdrawn from the very first moment of its existence from any direct deliberate attack. This is a fundamental right of the human person, which is of general value in the Christian conception of life; hence as valid for the life still hidden within the womb of the mother, as for the life already born and developing outside of her; as much opposed to direct abortion as to the direct killing of the child before, during or after its birth. *Whatever foundation there may be for the distinction between these various phases of the development of life* that is born or still unborn, in profane and ecclesiastical law, and as regards certain civil and penal consequences, all these cases involve a grave and unlawful attack upon the inviolability of human life. (Emphasis added)[22]

Seven years later Pius XII spoke to the International Association of Applied Psychology. He insisted that man is a person, a "self," from the *first* to the *last* moment of his life, even when he is not aware of his selfhood:

> Man is always a person, an "individual" distinct from all others, a "self" from the first to the last moment of his life, even when he is not conscious of it. We find, therefore, a certain difference between this point of view and the expressions of psychology . . .[23]

In the same context Pope Pius XII specifically referred to the twofold basis of value in human personhood: man's likeness to God, proceeding from the creative act (Creation), and his divine sonship in Christ, made known through revelation (Re-Creation).[24]

Pope John XXIII is remembered especially for *Mater et Magistra* which renewed the social justice principles of *Rerum Novarum* and *Quadragesimo Anno.* He spoke *there* of the dignity of the human person as "social by nature and raised to an order of existence that transcends and subdues nature."[25] Pope John likewise reaffirmed the sacredness of human life and the danger of weakening the community should this sacredness be compromised.[26]

Four years later, in solemn assembly, the Second Vatican Council promulgated its memorable document, *The Church in the Modern World (Gaudium et Spes).* Chapter Two, Part One, of that document contains a contemporary *Magna Carta* of human personhood:

> Every day human interdependence grows more tightly drawn and spreads by degrees over the whole world. As a result the common good, that is, the sum of those conditions of social life which allow social groups and their individual members relatively thorough and ready access to their own fulfillment, today takes on an increasingly universal complexion and consequently involves rights and duties with respect to the whole human race. Every social group must take account of the needs and the legitimate aspirations of other groups, and even of the general welfare of the entire human family.
>
> At the same time, however, there is a growing awareness of the exalted dignity proper to the human person, since he stands above all things, and his rights and duties are universal and inviolable. . . . Hence, the social order and its development must unceasingly work for the benefit of the human person if the disposition of affairs is to be subordinate to the personal realm and for man, and not man for the Sabbath.[27]
>
> Furthermore, whatever is opposed to life itself, such as any type of murder, genocide, abortion, euthanasia, or willful self-destruction, whatever violates the integrity of the human person, such as mutilation, torments inflicted on body or mind, . . . ; all these things and others of their like are infamies indeed. They poison human society, but they do more harm to those who practice them than those who suffer from the injury. Moreover, they are a supreme dishonor to the Creator.[28]
>
> Since all men possess a rational soul and are created in God's likeness, since they have the same nature and origin, have been redeemed by Christ, and enjoy the same divine calling and destiny, the basic equality of all must receive increasingly greater recognition.[29]

Seven years later, in December,1972, as the international movement for the legalization of abortion gathered momentum, in a vigorous address to the Society of Italian Catholic Jurists, Pope Paul VI insisted on the "personality" of the unborn child and the single, univocal vital process which begins at conception and culminates with birth:

> There is no doubt that this protection should start from conception—not with birth or with the attainment of adulthood. For conception

is the beginning of a single, univocal vital process which ends with the birth of a new human being.[30]

In the same context he added,

> The problem of abortion, as it is called, cannot be formulated solely in terms of an individualistic consideration of the woman; it must also be formulated in terms of the common good and, above all, in terms of the personality of the unborn child.[31]

Pope Paul went on to describe the mother-fetus relationship as a universal human value.[32] This universal human value found in the reciprocal rights and duties of the mother-child relationship could hardly be so described if the fetus were a non-person.

Six weeks later the U.S. Supreme Court issued its famous *Roe* v. *Wade* decision of January 22, 1973, which legalized the practice of abortion. This undoubtedly helped stimulate the thorough treatment of abortion in the "Declaration on Abortion" issued late the following year by the Sacred Congregation for the Doctrine of the Faith. In the section "Arguments from Reason", this document presents systematically the teaching of Pius XII and Paul VI as outlined above:

> The right to life is the primordial right of the human person. The person has other goods, some of them even more precious to him than life, but the right to life is the foundation and condition of all others. It is not within the competence of society or public authority, whatever its form, to give that right to some and take it away from others. Any such discrimination on grounds of race or sex, skin color or religion, is always unjust. The right to life does not derive from the favor of other human beings but exists prior to any such favor and must therefore be acknowledged as such. The denial of it is an injustice in the strict sense of the word.
>
> Discrimination based on the various stages of human life is no less inexcusable than discrimination on any other grounds. The right to life belongs intact to the elderly person, no matter how poor his health. It is not lost by the incurably ill. It belongs no less to the newborn child than to the mature adult. In fact, every human life must be respected from the moment the process of generation begins. For, as soon as the egg is fertilized, a life begins that belongs not to the father or mother but to the new living human being who now develops on his own account. He will never become human if he is not already human.
>
> Contemporary genetic science affords valuable confirmation of this point, which has indeed always been evident and does not depend in any way on solving the problem of the precise time of animation. Science has shown that from the very first moment this living being possesses a stable structure or genetic program; it is a human being,

an individual human being with all its characteristic traits already fixed. At the moment of fertilization the marvelous course of human life begins, even if each of the great powers by which that life is exercised requires time to become properly disposed and readied for action.[33]

The philosophical debate concerning the exact moment when the spiritual soul is infused, whether at conception or at some point early in fetal development, was not addressed definitively in the above document. However, the right to life, the "primordial right of the human person," *is* attributed to the newly-conceived zygote. The document argues that from conception the new being is already human and must be treated with the reverence given to human persons. The immediate infusion of the spiritual soul is considered at least probable and the contrary will never be established with certainty.[34]

The above outline of official Catholic statements over the past 25 years does not provide explicit references to fetal experimentation. But they indicate forcefully the contemporary insistence of the Catholic Church on the Biblical teaching about the beginning of personhood and the human dignity of the fetus. It seems obvious, therefore, that severe moral limits must be placed on non-therapeutic experimentation of children and fetuses. Pope Pius XII described eloquently the function of such moral limits in his 1952 address to the First International Congress of Histopathology:

> People will perhaps object that the ideas set forth here present a serious obstacle to scientific research and work. Nevertheless, the limits we have outlined are not by definition an obstacle to progress. The field of medicine cannot be different in this respect from other fields of man's research, investigations and work. The great moral demands force the impetuous flood of human thought and will to flow, like water from the mountains, into certain channels. They contain the flow to increase its efficiency and usefulness. They dam it so that it does not overflow and cause ravages that can never be compensated for by the special good it seeks. In appearance, moral demands are a brake. In fact, they contribute to the best and most beautiful of what man has produced for science, the individual and the community.[35]

Is this position of recent Popes about the value of the fetus from conception definitive Catholic teaching? Certainly it does not have the status of a defined dogma of faith and morals, but like the teaching of *Humanae Vitae* on contraception, remains open to modification by the teaching authority of the Church. Because it is not definitive it leaves room for further discussion and even responsible dissent by theologians. However, the consistency of development of thought on this question is impressive and it seems to rest on more fundamental grounds than the explicit condemnation of artificial contraception.

Protestant Theology from Luther to the Present on the Beginnings of Personhood

Early Protestant Views

As George Williams has shown, Luther and Calvin returned to the patristic tradition (especially as represented by St. Augustine) in their conviction that the fetus is the work of the Creator who has made man in His image and that abortion is a crime against the sovereignty of the Creator.[36] Dismissing the speculations of the scholastic theologians about delayed animation, they were content with the Biblical data which we have already summarized. Calvin found no difficulty in dealing with *Exodus* 21:22, and noted that if a "man's home is his castle," so the fetus has a right to protection in its natural home, the maternal womb.

Granted the fetus' right to protection, the Protestant theologians had also to wrestle with the conflict situations and did so by a route different than casuistic distinctions used by their Catholic confreres. They admitted exceptions to any rule formulated by theologians or by church officials, and yet attempted to protect the dignity of the fetus by reference to Biblical values.

Such Protestant teaching is very clear and forceful in writings of many of the outstanding theologians of this century.[37] Thus Karl Barth, an outstanding contemporary representative of the Calvinist tradition, raises the question of whether abortion is licit and then answers:

> The fact that a definite NO must be the presupposition of all further discussion cannot be contested, least of all today. The question arises, however, how this NO is to be established and stated if it is to be a truly effective NO. In face of the wicked violation of the sanctity of human life which is always seriously at issue in abortion and which is always present, if it is carried out thoughtlessly and callously, the only thing which can help is the power of a wholly new and radical feeling of awe at the mystery of all human life as this is commanded by God as its Creator, Giver and Lord. . . . The command of God is based on His grace. He summons man to freedom in which he may live instead of having to live. At root, the man who thinks he must live cannot and will not respect life, whether his own or that of others, far less the life of an unborn child . . . Those who live by mercy will always be disposed to practice mercy, especially to a human being which is so dependent on the mercy of others as the unborn child.[38]

Similarly, the martyr Dietrich Bonhoeffer, perhaps made sensitive to the value of human life by the rise of the Nazi ideology, wrote:

> Marriage involves acknowledgement of the right of life that is to come into being, a right which is not subject to the disposal of the married couple. Unless this right is acknowledged as a matter of pinciple, marriage ceases to be marriage and becomes a mere

liaison. Acknowledgement of this right means making way for the free creative power of God which can cause new life to proceed from this marriage according to His will. Destruction of the embryo in the mother's womb is a violation of the right to live which God has bestowed upon this nascent life. To raise the question whether we are here concerned already with a human being or not is merely to confuse the issue. The simple fact is that God certainly intended to create a human being and this nascent human being has been deliberately deprived of his life. And that is nothing but murder.[39]

Again, Helmut Thielicke, perhaps the leading Lutheran ethicist today, writes:

> The genesis of human life is a sacrosanct domain which dare not be invaded by human hands or "rationalized," that is, subject to utilitarian considerations. And this inviolability over and against any pragmatic intervention follows not only from the order of creation, the miracle of which has actualized itself and the violation of which must be atoned for, but also from the order of redemption, just as surely as Christ has bought man "with a price" and bestows upon him an "alien dignity" *(dignitas aliena).* This "alien dignity" expresses the fact that it is not man's or his value for producing "good works," his functional proficiency, his pragmatic utility that gives him his dignity, but rather what God has "spent upon him," the sacrificial love which God has invested in him (*Deut.* 7:7 f.).[40]

Nor is this view of fetal dignity now obsolete among Protestant theologians. Very much the same position is taken in current writings by Paul Ramsey and by Albert Outler.[41] It should be noted that all these writers (with the possible exception of Bonhoeffer) admit exceptions to the law against abortion in concrete situations (especially where the life of the mother is endangered), but they are emphatic in insisting on the human dignity of the fetus.

Contemporary Protestant Thought

Since 1950, however, a new trend has appeared in Protestant thinking in the United States on this question. It is put very well by J. Robert Nelson, Dean of Boston University School of Theology, in an article, "What does Theology Say about Abortion?"[42] He introduces a new note by distinguishing two senses of the word "life":

1. *Bios* or biological life; and
2. *Zoe* or properly human life which involves interpersonal relations.

He then argues that the process of human development from conception to birth is a gradual advance from merely biological life to fully human life. Consequently, in a decision about abortion, it is necessary to take into account the fact that the mother has life in the full sense of *zoe,* while the fetus has this only in an increasing degree as it approaches term.[43]

It appears that a new element in Protestant thinking is the basic notion that the fetus is not yet a person, but only on the way to personhood. Hence, its dignity or value is comparable not only to the life of the mother (as the older Protestant writers had admitted), but to other less fundamental values (e.g., the physical or mental health of the mother, the economic and educative welfare of the existing family, etc.), so that abortion is justifiable not only in the extremity but in many life situations. Thus on October 14, 1974, the Seventh General Convention of the American Lutheran Church adopted by a vote of 500 to 379 a statement "Christian Counseling on Abortion," which is to a substantial degree compatible with the classical attitude, but which adds to this several significant sentences about the occasional need to terminate a developing life.[44] A similar thought is found in an earlier official statement published by the Eighth General Synod of the United Church of Christ, which called for "the repeal of all legal prohibitions of physician-performed abortions."[45] This trend has been general among the more liberal Protestant churches, and although the Evangelical churches have generally supported the former position, in their ranks, too, questions are raised mainly on the grounds that there is no clear Biblical commandment forbidding abortion.[46]

Other recent writers, e.g., Joseph Fletcher, Ronald M. Green and H. Tristram Engelhardt, Jr., have argued for this point of view, attempting to establish a distinction between child and fetus in terms of interpersonal relationships.[47] As was mentioned in the Chapter III discussion of delayed hominization, some contemporary philosophers restrict personhood to those fetuses or infants already functioning in a uniquely human way.

However, it seems that a new element influencing Protestant theology has been a new attitude toward *pastoral experience.* Rachel Conrad Wahlberg, reporting on the conference held in 1973 at Southern Methodist University in Dallas summarized the discussion by saying:

> Those who are not involved personally with an unwanted pregnancy tend to discuss the philosophical, medical or moral questions. Those who face nine months of pregnancy and 15 to 20 years of child-raising are more concerned with the immediate crisis.[48]

And Constance Parvey, writing in *Dialogue,* said: "The basic question revolves around the social consequences: *'What actually happens to the women and to babies who are unwanted?'.*"[49] These women are demanding that theologians look at the problem more in terms of the experience of the unwilling mother and the unwanted child. In 1967, a group of activist ministers in New York City, appalled by the problems of poor mothers, and the unjust laws which permitted the middle and upper classes to solve their problems by abortion and which denied this to poor women with far fewer options, founded the Clergy Consultative Service on Abortion and began to work actively for a repeal of laws restricting abortions. They were followed by many liberal and socially activist clergy throughout the country.[50] The experience of these zealous and compassionate ministers seems to have had a widespread effect on Protestant opinion.

It should not be overlooked that this shift toward a "theology of experience" and a "theology of liberation" which first begins by asking: "How does this problem look from the viewpoint of the woman driven to consider abortion?" is significant and valuable. A truly pastoral theology is not just one which draws pastoral applications from abstract principles, but one which also looks carefully into the real experiences of people in conflict situations and uses principles validated by pastoral experience. However, to date, such a new theology of the experience of the abortion situation (fetus and the pregnant woman) is still not fully developed, and what has come forth is, thus far, largely rhetoric.[51]

Protestant-Catholic Divergences and Rapprochement

Attitudes on Original Sin and Baptism.

There were important differences between the Reformers and the Catholics on the existential condition of the unborn child as the result of original sin. Following Augustine, all agreed that the fetus is affected by original sin from conception. The Reformers saw these effects as "total depravity"; the Catholics took a more moderate view. Moreover, Luther returned to the view of Tertullian and the earlier Augustine, which is called "paternal traducianism," i.e., that the human soul infected by sin is transmitted to the fetus by the father's semen, while the Catholics generally held that the soul incurred original sin from the flesh at the moment of its immediate creation and infusion by God into the body of the fetus produced by the parents. This traducianism, however, found little acceptance by later Protestant divines, although Father Albert Plé has recently raised the question as to whether this old theory is still a significant influence in both Protestant and Catholic thinking.[52]

What was more significant for the issue in question, however, was the difference in attitude toward infant baptism as the remedy of original sin. Catholic theologians generally held that sacramental baptism was the sole means of salvation for the child before the age of reason, when a personal act of faith and conversion became possible, although Cardinal Cajetan, among the first of the commentators on the *Summa Theologica* of St. Thomas, and others believed that the prayers of the parents or the Church might attain this goal in anticipation of baptism. However, after the Council of Trent, the common opinion and practice of the Roman Catholic Church followed the stricter Augustinian view, mitigated by the "limbo theory" of Aquinas, that the souls of the unbaptized were not damned, but consigned to a state of "natural beatitude" instead of the "beatific vision."

Luther, in spite of his Augustinianism, taught a view similar to that of Cajetan. Calvin, on the other hand, went even beyond Augustine in holding that the salvation or damnation of the fetus was predetermined by God's predestination anterior even to the creation of the soul. Thus, while Luther and Calvin accepted infant baptism, it lacked for them the crucial practical importance attributed to it by Roman Catholics. George Williams (see footnote # 36) may be right in thinking that Catholic opinion was pushed to uniformity in reaction to the downgrading of the importance of infant baptism by the Reformers.

Conflict Situations and Pastoral Experience

A final important difference between Protestants and Catholics was in their manner and method of dealing with *pastoral problems of conflicting values.* In the period following Trent, there developed among Catholics the type of special "moral theology" concerned with "cases of conscience."[53] The basic rule of this theology was that it is never ethical deliberately to act (or to omit decision) in a "state of *practical* doubt" as to the morality of the action (or of an omission). The task of the confessor or counselor, therefore, was to assist the client to resolve his or her doubts of conscience and to arrive at a prudent, or practically certain decision. Ordinarily this required the counselor to instruct the client in the moral law as authentically interpreted by the Church or by the common teaching of moral experts. At times, however, the counselor was obliged to "leave the penitent in good faith" when such instruction might actually hinder the client in resolving his doubts of conscience and acting in accordance with conscience. In instructing the client the counselor was to advise him as to the maximum freedom allowed within the law as interpreted by theologians, according to the principle of *probabilism* by which it was permitted to follow more lenient interpretations or applications of a law, providing these had at least "solid probability." The exception to this was in matters where the risk of salvation, human life, or the validity of the sacraments were at stake.

With the Protestant view of the fallen state of Man, who, even after justification, remains *simul justus et peccator* (simultaneously just and a sinner), the notion that the conscience can never be free of doubt seemed preposterous. Peace of mind comes not from the consciousness that what we are doing is simply and unambiguously the *right* thing to do, but rather from our *faith* that God, because of the Cross of Christ, will forgive whatever is of sin in all that we do.

The Catholic system of "casuistry" was generally rejected by the Protestant tradition, which tended to emphasize *the ambiguity* of all moral decision in this sinful world. Thus it is typical of human decisions that they involve a conflict of values in which, at best, man chooses the "lesser evil and the greater good."[54] Roman Catholic casuistry thus tends to appear to Protestants not only as dishonest, since it cloaks moral ambiguity with an appearance of innocence, but as dangerous because it hides from the Christian his need for forgiveness in all that he does, and blinds him with self-righteousness. Rather it is better to confess that in all our decisions an element of compromise with a sinful world remains.[55]

In both the Roman Catholic and the Protestant traditions, it has been admitted that there are certain situations involving both the rights of the mother and of the fetus in which it is difficult to find a reasonable solution. These arise precisely because of the dignity of the fetus. But the *rationale of the solution* is different in the two traditions. The Catholic seeks to find a solution which is strictly *consistent* with the moral law by means of careful distinctions between "direct" and "indirect," the "double effects of an action," etc. The Protestant believes it is necessary to admit that *no* solution consistent with the moral law may be possible, considering the sinful condition of this world, and therefore, we must make the most prudent decision possible while asking for forgiveness of God. This is not the place to discuss the roots of these two positions, but it is important to see that two moral methodologies are at work, and that they should not be compared in terms of "permissiveness." In fact, each one in different circumstances yields the more rigorous conclusion.

The result in the present case has generally been that Roman Catholic theology has become more and more rigorous in its consistent belief that it is "never licit to take the life of the innocent," and hence is opposed to any direct destruction of the fetus, even to save the life of the mother.[56] At the same time Catholic theologians have elaborated casuistic distinctions to solve conflict situations remaining consistent with official teaching. Protestant theology, on the other hand, has sought solutions to these same cases by another route, admitting exceptions to any rule formulated by theologians or by church officials, and yet attempting to protect the dignity of the fetus by reference to Biblical values.

Convergences

Evidence of the stirrings of a movement toward a Catholic-Protestant rapprochement may be seen in the following reflections. While the classical Protestant position in its doctrine of original sin differs somewhat from the Catholic tradition, it joins the latter at the level of Biblical teaching and in its common acceptance of the patristic tradition on the sacred character of fetal life. That is, both Catholic and Protestant theology affirm the immediate relation of every human being to God, and therefore its value, from the beginning of its existence as a unique individual created by God in His image and redeemed by the death and resurrection of His Son Jesus Christ.

The major divergence with regard to the pastoral solution of conflict situations is today beginning to be overcome in the recognition by both traditions of the fact that, since the late Middle Ages, Christian ethics has been unduly voluntaristic (and hence legalistic) in its orientation. On the part of Catholics this is currently leading to a re-examination of the manner in which conflict situations are resolved without lapsing into mere "situationism."[57]

This trend predisposes Catholic thinking to a greater awareness of and sensitivity to the experience of the victim (i.e., the mother) of the conflict situation. At the same time, a number of Catholic theologians are willing to speculate about the possibility of locating hominization at some point later than conception.[58] Others believe that the casuistic method of probabilism can be applied to justify abortion in some cases.[59] These efforts have not yet markedly affected the official Catholic teaching, and are perhaps mistaken, but they are proof that responsible Catholic theologians are painstakingly testing every facet of the Catholic tradition and contemporary experience.

The Protestant view is similar. Thus one has only to read recent essays by James M. Gustafson, Gabriel Fackre, and Paul Ramsey to see that these theologians have developed the classical position of their own tradition in a similar manner.[60]

The essential point is that, there is a common rejection of those arguments in the abortion controversy which concentrate simply, as did the Supreme Court decision, on the rights of the mother. All are agreed that the fetus must be an object of serious Christian concern and care, which means that the problem of determining the way and the time that human personhood begins must be a subject of continuing scientific study and careful philosophical interpretation. However, respect for the unborn does not depend on a certain determination of this issue, since the Christian theology sees the whole process in terms of God's creative activity and the goal of salvation.

Moreover, all these theologians insist on two points about legislation with respect to fetal care: (1) The civil law is *not* the ultimate determinative of moral responsiblity; (2) The law does, however, have an educative function. Consequently, all are concerned to arrive at legislation which (a) will protect freedom and pluralism; and, (b) will provide better alternatives than abortion for the solution of human problems.

In the matter of fetal experimentation, therefore, it seems that the Christian churches can bear a common witness to the need for protection of unborn human life. In this area the conflict with the rights of the mother is ordinarily not present. The primary issue is whether restrictions on experimentation designed to protect fetal life may unduly hamper scientific progress that will be to the advantage of future life. Generally, Christians are here united in the conviction that present life cannot simply be sacrificed to the future, but must be confident that creative scientists will be able to find other ways to carry on effective research.

Summary

While the Bible does not supply proof-texts which specifically treat dilemmas related to embryological questions, it does provide a profound teaching on the origin of every human person. Throughout the Old Testament there is a growing emphasis on the I-Thou relationship established by the Creator with each of His human creatures from the outset of their existence. At the same time a similar relationship is constituted among all members of the human community. In the New Testament, the Incarnation of the Divine Son as Jesus Christ provided the archetype by which Christians understood their own personal relation with the Father, a relationship celebrated in baptism, but initiated in grace by the divine call which brought them into existence as human beings.

In the patristic period of the Christian Church, abortion was generally rejected as a form of infanticide. Medieval theologians occupied with the classification of sins, and influenced by Greek philosophy, took the view that abortion was not technically homicide, although it was a grave sin against nature, even if it took place during the earliest period of fetal life. In the Renaissance and Reformation periods moral theologians, with the tolerance of church authorities, permitted some forms of therapeutic abortion. However, with the rise of modern embryology and a greater concern for consistency in church discipline, the Holy See took a strict anti-abortion position, confirmed recently by Vatican II. Nevertheless, some Catholic theologians continue to argue for more lenient views.

At first sight, there seems to be great divergence between the official Catholic stand and that of Protestant theologians. However, on closer examination, it is evident that the Protestant tradition in this matter is much the same as the Catholic. The practical divergence in dealing with hardship cases comes largely from the difference between the casuistic methodology familiar to Catholics, and the Protestant emphasis on the moral ambiguity of human decisions. It seems, therefore, that it should be possible by honest and charitable dialogue gradually to increase the area of consensus based on fundamental Christian principles held in common. It would seem that with regard to the ethics of fetal experimentation, this agreement should be relatively easy.

CHAPTER IV Footnotes

1. Pius XII, "Modern Technology and Peace" (1953 Christmas Address), *Major Addresses of Pope Pius XII,* Vol. II, Yzermans, V. A., editor, St. Paul: North Central Pub. Co., 1961, p. 177.
2. The question of the *manner* in which the human soul is created by God is discussed at some length by Robert North, S.J. in his *Teilhard and the Creation of the Soul,* Milwaukee: The Bruce Publishing Co., 1967. See also Schoonenbert, Piet, S.J., *The Christ,* New York: Herder and Herder, 1971.
3. Pius XII, *Humani Generis,* New York: Paulist Press, 1950, # 62. See Fr. North's discussion regarding a more nuanced reading of this passage: *Op. cit.,* p. 206-7.
4. Yet the difficulty clearly stated by Fr. North should not be overlooked: "Sertillanges, Rahner, and almost all theologians who have recently talked about the problem deplore the evil of a terminology which makes it appear that the parents produce one part of the child and God produces a different part . . . Human parents, with God's creative concurrence, produce a human being, body and soul." *Op. cit.,* p. 257, 259.
5. See especially Wolff, Hans Walter, *Anthropology of the Old Testament,* Philadelphia: Fortress Press, 1973, All Biblical quotations are from *The New American Bible.*
6. According to Martin Buber, the Jewish philosopher, the Semite saw God and the individual in an "I-Thou" relationship.
7. Stamm, Johann J., "Name", *Encyclopedia Judaica,* 12: col. 803-806, esp. 804.
8. See Wolff, *op. cit.,* pp. 96 and 10-24.
9. See Dubarle, Andre-Marie, *The Biblical Doctrine of Original Sin,* New York: Herder

and Herder, 1964, pp. 23 ff.

10. Rabinnical decisions do permit abortion in certain difficult cases, especially in those in which there is danger to the life of the mother and which do not recognize the child as legally a human person "until the head emerges." Yet these casuistic decisions have no foundation in the Biblical text, except a single verse, *Exodus* 21:22: "When men have a fight and hurt a pregnant woman, so that she suffers a miscarriage, but no further injury, the guilty one shall be fined as much as the woman's husband demands of him, and he shall pay in the presence of the judges. But if injury ensues, you shall give life for life."

    Rabbinic tradition generally understood this text to mean that since for the life of a fetus, only a money fine is prescribed, rather than "a life for a life", the fetus cannot be a person in the same sense as the woman for whose mortal injury "a life for a life" is required. However, this is an archaic law, exactly paralleled in the Code of Hammurabi. It deals not with deliberate or direct abortion, but with an accidental or indirect abortion and is concerned with the damages due to the husband for losses suffered to his property (wife and child). The immediately preceding verse 21 gives the rule that punishes a master who kills a slave with death, yet provides that if the slave survives the beating "one or two days", the master "is not to be punished, since the slave is his own property". Clearly, this crude justice is at a much less developed level of religious sensitivity than the view of man presented by the Yahwist, the writers of the Psalms, and the Prophets. This was evidently felt by later Judaism, since the translators of the Septuagint introduced in these verses a distinction between the "unformed" and the "formed foetus", and Philo says the same in *De Specialibus Legibus* 3:108-109. In the deutero-canonical *Book of Wisdom,* Solomon is portrayed as saying:

    > I, too, am a mortal man, the same as all the rest,
    > and a descendant of the first man formed of earth.
    > And in my mother's womb I was molded into flesh in a
    > ten-months' period—body and blood,
    > from the seed of man, and the pleasure that
    > accompanies marriage.
    > And I, too, when born, inhaled the common air,
    > and fell upon the kindred earth;
    > wailing, I uttered that first sound common to all.
    > In swaddling clothes and with constant care
    > I was nurtured.
    > For no king has any different origin or birth,
    > but one is the entry into life for all;
    > and in one same way they leave it.
    >
    > (7:1-6)

    Thus, Alexandrine Judaism, perhaps disturbed by the callous attitude of the pagans toward children, tended to emphasize the sacredness even of unborn life. Note that the rabbis, in taking a more permissive attitude toward abortion, did not view it lightly. They were not approving it as such, but seeking by a legal casuistry to solve limit-cases in which there was a conflict of rights; and they naturally used the single Scriptural text that gave some legal guidance, rather than seek out deeper theological principles. (See Elon, Menachen, "Abortion", *Encyclopedia Judaica,* I, col. 98-101.)

11. See Brown, Raymond E., *The Virginal Conception and the Bodily Resurrection of Jesus,* New York: Paulist Press, 1973; Laurentin, Rene, *Structure et Theologie de Luc I-II,* Paris: Gabalda, 1964, and *Jesus au Temple,* Paris: Gabalda, 1966; Feuillet, A., *Jesus et sa Mere d'apres les recits Lucaniens de l'enfance et d'apres Saint Jean,* Paris: Gabalda, 1974; Humenay, Robert L., "The Place of Mary in Luke: A Look at Modern Biblical Criticism", *American Ecclesiastical Review,* May, 1974; Ryder, A., "Parents' Faith and Baptism", *Clergy Review,* March, 1969; Rahner, Karl, "The Immaculate Conception in our Life", *Theological Investigations,* vol. 3, 1967.

12. God has intervened in human history in the very begetting of great leaders of the Chosen People. It is clear that Luke, in Chapters 1-2, is strongly influenced by the account of the begetting of the patriarch Isaac (Genesis 18:9-15), the judge, Samson (*Judges* 13), the first of the prophets, Samuel (*I Samuel* 1-2:11), and the great prophet of the Exile and the figure of the Suffering Servant, Jeremiah (1:5). In all but the last account, there is an angelic annunciation to sterile parents who have prayed for a child in a faith that looks toward the salvation of their people; then God's promise

that this child will have a mission in the work of salvation. This list should probably also include the wonderful preservation of Moses as an infant, and the prophecy of Isaiah of the coming birth of Immanuel (*Exodus* 2 and *Isaiah* 7:14). Luke places the conception of John the Baptizer and finally of Jesus, the Saviour Himself, as the completion of this same age-old pattern. For Matthew (1:22-23), this is the fulfillment of the Immanuel prophecy as well.

13. Feuillet, *op. cit.,* p. 17-29. For the theological implications, see Congar, Yves, The Mystery of the Temple, Westminster, Maryland, 1962. In a still more profound sense, of course, Jesus Himself is the New Temple by reason of the fact that He is made flesh through Mary (*John* 2:21).
14. Noonan, John T., Jr., editor, *The Morality of Abortion: Legal and Historical Perspectives,* Cambridge, Massachusetts: Harvard University Press, 1970, pp. 1-59. See also his "The Catholic Church and Abortion", *Dublin Review,* 261, Winter, 1967-68, pp. 300-345, and his *Contraception: A History of its Treatment by the Catholic Theologians and Canonists,* Harvard University Press, 1965. For other historical summaries, see Granfield, David, *The Abortion Decision,* New York: Doubleday, 1969, pp. 43-62; Callahan, Daniel, *Abortion: Law, Choice, and Morality,* New York: Macmillan, 1970, c. xii, pp. 409-447; Grisez, Germain, *Abortion: The Myths, the Realities, and the Arguments,* New York: Corpus Books, 1970, c. IV., "Religious Views of Abortion", pp. 117-184; Connery, John P., "Fetal Life—Is It Human?: An Historical Perspective", *Theology Digest,* 22, Spring, 1974, and his review of Grisez' book in Theological Studies, 21, 1970, pp. 170-176; Curran, Charles, *New Perspectives in Moral Theology,* Notre Dame, Indiana: Fides, 1974, pp. 175-179; and Dedek, John F., *Contemporary Medical Ethics,* New York: Sheed and Ward, 1975, pp. 109-120. Also on the background in the Jewish tradition, see Feldman, David, *Birth Control in Jewish Law,* New York: New York University Press, 1968, and Elon, Menachon, "Abortion", *Encyclopedia Judaica,* Vol. 1, col. 98-101.
15. On the origin and significance of this commandment (which was probably taken over by Christians from a Jewish source), see Audet, J. P., *La Didache: Instructions des Apotres,* Paris: Gabalda, 1958, pp. 288 ff.
16. Tertullian, *Apologeticum ad Nationes,* 1.15, quoted by Noonan, *The Morality of Abortion,* p. 12. Undoubtedly, Tertullian's views are somewhat colored by his traducianism; see Appendix I, n.4. Nevertheless, his position is typical of this period and affirmed by non-traducianists.
17. The history of this is well discussed by Dedek, *loc. cit.* Dedek himself concludes: "In summary, therefore, we should say that although the majority of Catholic theologians still support the teaching of the Magisterium, which absolutely proscribes all direct abortion no matter what the reason, there is a sizeable and growing number of contemporary Catholic theologians who are arguing that there are some exceptions to this general rule . . . Contemporary theologians are only returning to an earlier theological position, saying that the prohibition of abortion is not an absolute one. Ordinarily, the purposeful destruction of a fetus is morally wrong. But exceptions to this rule have to be made when a proportionate value, another life or its moral equivalent, is at stake." (p. 31) However, the main ground for Dedek's defense of the probability of the moral view is based on biological arguments for delayed hominization. In Appendix I, it is argued that such biological arguments are so weak as to be incapable of grounding a practical moral probability.
18. See Appendix I, n. 3 for references.
19. *"Declaration on Abortion", Origins, 4*(25): 385-392, Dec. 12, 1974; See also, *The Pope Speaks,* Vol. 19, No. 3, Winter, 1975, pp. 250-262, p. 256.
20. Noonan, *The Morality of Abortion, op. cit.,* pp. 36-7.
21. Allocution to Midwives, October 29, 1951 in *The Human Body: Papal Teachings,* edited by Monks of Solesmes, Boston: Daughters of St. Paul Press, 1960, p. 150.
22. Pius XII, "Moral Questions Affecting Married Life", Washington, 1951, p. 26. See *Acta Apostolicae Sedis,* 43, 1951, p. 857.
23. "The Human Personality", address of Pope Pius XII to Thirteenth Congress of the International Association of Applied Psychology, April 10, 1958 in *Major Addresses of Pope Pius XII,* Vol. 1, Yzermans, V. A., editor, St. Paul: North Central Publishing Co., 1961, p. 436.
24. *Ibid.*

25. *Mater et Magistra,* # 219.
26. "Indeed, all must regard the life of man as sacred, since from its inception, it required the action of God the Creator. Those who depart from this plan of God not only offend His divine majesty and dishonor themselves and the human race, but they also weaken the inner fibre of the commonwealth." *Ibid.,* #194.
27. "The Church Today", *Documents of Vatican II,* Abbott, Walter M., S.J., editor, New York: Guild Press, 1966, p. 225, paragraph # 26.
28. *Ibid.,* pp. 226-7, paragraph # 27.
29. *Ibid.,* p. 227, paragraph #29.
30. Pope Paul VI, "The Right to be Born", (address to Society of Italian Catholic Jurists, December 9, 1972), *The Pope Speaks,* Vol. 17, No. 4, 1973, p. 334.
31. *Ibid.,* p. 335.
32. *Ibid.,* p. 335: "Implicit in this vocation, and destined to assume concrete form, is the first and most fundamental of those relationships that make up the human personality; the relationship between this one new human being and this one woman who is its mother. Now to say *relationship* is to say *right.* To talk about a fundamental human relationship is to talk about a *universal human value* which deserves to be protected as part of the equally universal common good, since every individual is first of all and constitutively *born of woman.*" (italics not added)
33. "Declaration on Abortion", *The Pope Speaks,* Vol. 19, No. 3, Winter, 1975, pp. 250-262, pp. 256-7.
34. See the footnote quoted above as appended to this passage in *The Pope Speaks, ibid.,* p. 256, and see Appendix I which critiques the Theory of Delayed Hominization.
35. "Moral Limits of Medical Research", see Yzermans, *op. cit.,* p. 234 (see footnote #23 above).
36. Williams, George, "Religious Residues and Presuppositions in the American Debate on Abortion", *Theological Studies* 31:10-75, 1970. It is especially helpful as a history of Protestant opinion.
37. Smith, Harmon L., *Ethics and the New Medicine,* Nashville: Abingdon, 1970, pp. 17-54, surveys several of these and attempts to undermine their arguments by what seems to be rather specious reasoning.
38. Church Dogmatics, Vol. III, Part Four, pp. 417 ff. Edinburgh: T & T Clark Ltd., *A. T. MacKay et al,* translators, 1961.
39. *Ethics,* New York: Macmillan Co., pp. 175-6. Bonhoeffer, footnote #12, p. 177, even refers to the Catholic refusal to save the life of the mother by destroying the fetus with seeming approval, while Barth misunderstood this, thinking preference was given by Catholics to the life of the mother.
40. *The Ethics of Sex,* New York: Harper and Row, 1964, p. 231.
41. For a critique and a bibliography of Ramsey's writings on this subject, see Curran, Charles E., *Politics, Medicine and Christian Ethics: A Dialogue with Paul Ramsey,* Philadelphia: Fortress Press, pp. 114-135. For a summary of Outler's views, see Outler, Albert C., "Beginnings of Personhood: Theological Considerations", *Perkins Journal of Theology* 27:2, Fall, 1973.
42. *Christian Century* 90:124-8, January 31, 1973.
43. Nelson applies this quite restrictively, however: "Christians would never think of the fetus, at whatever stage of development, as a disposable 'thing', nor would they have so strong a fixation on the preservation of the fetus 'at all costs' that they would be callous to either the pregnant woman's *zoe* or to the well-being of society. Then they could respect fully the rights of women without being coerced into thinking women are always right. Then they could have the perception needed to resist the notion that an 'unwanted child' had better not have been born. And, very important, they could see that a battle for the 'rights of the unborn' is only half a war against inhumanity - since the other half, which has equal claim on them, is the hard social and legislative struggle to secure and realize the rights of both the bearers and the born for a good life." (p. 128)
44. "The position taken by the American Lutheran Church is a pro-life position. It looks in awe at the mystery of procreation and at the processes through which a human being develops, matures, and dies. It takes seriously the right of developing life to be born. It takes into account the rights of the already born to their health, their individuality, and the wholeness of their lives. It allows the judgment that, all pertinent factors

responsibly considered, the developing life may need to be terminated in order to defend the health and wholeness of persons already present and already participating in relationships and responsibilities of life." Office of Research Analysis, The American Lutheran Church, 422 South Fifth Street, Minneapolis, Minnesota 55415.

45. "An ethical view does not require an *undifferentiated* concern for life. It places peculiar value upon *personal* life and upon the *quality* of life, both actual and potential. In that light, it is understandable that today an increasing number of persons find it difficult, if not impossible, to attribute anything more than the *potentiality* of human personhood to the embryo in its *early* stages. The implication is that factors other than its existence may appropriately be given equal or greater weight at this time - the welfare of the whole family, its economic condition, the age of the parents, their view of the optimum number of children consonant with their resources and the pressures of population, their vocational and social objectives, for example. On the other hand, many would agree that during the late months of a normal pregnancy, life should not be interrupted except for the most serious reasons, such as the physical or mental health of the mother, abnormality or disease of the fetus, incest, or rape. This distinction is of the greatest importance. Individuals contemplating an abortion should make a responsible decision early, certainly within the first two or three months." *Social Action* 38:9-12, S., 1971.

46. This is the argument of C. E. Cerling, Jr. in "Abortion and Contraception in Scripture", *Christian Scholar's Review* 2:42-58, Fall, 1971. Cerling concludes that "the fetus is an emerging entity, immeasurably valuable at conception and becoming increasingly valuable as the date of its birth approaches." (p. 58) Also, Bruce Waltke, in "Old Testament and Birth Control", *Christianity Today* 17:6-9, March 16, 1972, refutes these views by trying to show that *Exodus* 21:22 refers to premature birth and not to miscarriage. A money penalty, therefore, is due the father in payment of the risk of premature birth. But if either fetus or mother dies, the penalty is "life for a life."

47. The most systematic effort to argue for this view is that of Joseph Fletcher who at first proposed 15 positive and 5 negative "indicators of humanhood" and then refined these to four: (1) Subjectivity, or self-awareness; (2) Human relationships; (3) Euphoria (as in the retarded but "happy" child; (4) Neocortical function. See "Indicators of Humanhood: A Tentative Profile of Man," *Hastings Center Report,* November, 1972, and "Four Indicators of Humanhood—The Inquiry Matures", *ibid.,* December 1974, with replies in correspondence, April, 1975. Oddly, Fletcher at this point returns to a purely biological criterion, namely, neocortical function which he sees as the necessary basis of the other indicators.

However, others more philosophically inclined have tried to develop the notion of personhood as conferred through interpersonal relations, arguing that this does not necessarily prove too much by also validating infanticide. Thus, Ronald M. Green, making use of a "social contract" type of ethical theory (similar to the thinking of Baier, Gert, Richards, Gewrith, and especially Rawls), says that "The issue of abortion . . . comes down to the question of whether rational agents could find it rational in the circumstances of moral choice to confer rights on the fetus, and if so, the nature and extent of these rights." See "Conferred Rights and the Fetus", *Journal of Religious Ethics* 2:55-83, Spring, 1974, with the response of James Childress, *ibid.* 2:77-84. Also see Green's "Abortion and Promise-Keeping", *Christianity and Crisis* 27:109-113, May 15, 1967.

He argues further that rational agents reasonably confer human rights on all other rational agents, since only thus is non-coercive social peace possible. It is reasonable also that they confer such rights on infants, because of our sympathetic feelings for them, and on the insane and senile since we fear that we may someday share their fate. But it seems unreasonable for rational agents to give up the right to abort the fetus by conferring on it human rights, since we do not sympathize with an entity that has none or minimal feelings, and we have no fear of ever sharing their lot!

Similar, if less harshly stated, reasons are given by H. Tristram Engelhardt, Jr. a philosopher and a physician specializing in medical ethics, in "Beginnings of Personhood: Philosophical Considerations", *Perkins Journal of Theology* 27:2, Fall, 1973. He argues that human personhood is defined by "autonomous action, self-awareness, self-determination." This is not identical with human biological life, as is evident from the fact of "brain-death" in a comatose human being who no longer is alive as a person, but who remains biologically alive. For Englehardt, the life process is continuous from one human generation to the next and there is no point at which from a biological point of view we can say that one human life begins (an argument that recalls Luther's traducianism). Consequently, the "fetus is valuable to others but not to itself" (p. 23) and this value is only for what it may become, and is relative to the persons who value or dis-value it. On the other hand, this does not conclude to the lawfulness of infanticide, because the infant is treated by others only *as if* it were a person. It is really hard to believe that this kind of argument, which seems like a reversion to Hobbes, is likely to be of much comfort to Christian theologians. Vernard Eller seems to have the better of the argument when, in answer to Joseph Fletcher, he points out that (as Barth and Bonhoeffer had already pointed out) it is not essential to settle whether the conceptus *is* a person, but whether it is "going to be a *particular* person." Contraception prevents birth, but not the birth of any particular, unique being; but abortion is the "violent interdiction of a definite person who is definitely on the way." See "Let's Get Honest About Abortion", *Christian Century* 92:16-18, January 18, 1974.

48. "Abortion: Decisions to Live With", *Christian Century* 90:691-3, June 27, 1973.

49. "Abortion", *Dialogue* 11:304-307, Autumn, 1972. Answered by C. Jack Eichorst, *ibid.* 12:62-65, Winter 1973 and Leonard Klein, *ibid.* 12:142-147, Spring, 1973.

50. Howard Moody, one of the leaders of the movement, says that they took their stand on three principles: (1) self-determination of women; (2) the unborn's chances for happy life; (3) the need for population control. See "Abortion: Women's Rights and the Legal Problem", *Theology Today* 28:337-346, October, 1971.

    The tragic aspect of this well-intentioned effort was that this counselling tended to become simply a referral service to compliant doctors, and with the Supreme Court decision, the movement declined. Thus, the Chicago Clergy Consultation reported that it interviewed about 150 women a week and 77% of these elected abortion and were referred to a doctor. (See Parsons, E. Spencer, "Abortion: Private and Public Concern", *Criterion* 10:13-16, Winter, 1971.) There were second thoughts about it, like about so many enthusiastic movements of the '60's. Thus, C. Eric Lincoln, Professor of Sociology at Union Theological Seminary in New York, in an article, "Why I Reversed My Stand on Laissez-faire Abortion", writes:

    > My original position was largely motivated by an interpretation of sectarian dogma which seemed at the time anachronistic and repressive. My vision was of occasional individuals caught up in circumstances so overwhelming and so devastating in potential as to warrant so drastic a procedure as the interruption of life. . . . I was not prepared for the bloodletting which has, in fact, ensued . . . I, for one, am sick of bloodletting - in the streets, on the battlefield, and in the safe, asceptic privacy of a doctor's office.

    (See *Christian Century* 90:77-79, April 25, 1973.) Not all Protestant liberals identified with Moody's position. See Dyck, Arthur J., "Perplexities of the Would-be Liberal in Abortion", *Journal of Reproductive Medicine* 8:351-54, June, 1972.

51. For example, Howard Moody, writing in "Church, State, and the Rights of Conscience", speaks in the following terms:

    > Only the fanatic's overzealousness could bring the right-to-lifers to believe that all women should be compelled by a compulsory child-bearing law to believe and act as they do. Any religiously and morally sensitive person should be able to see that these restrictive laws are one of the last and the most formidable blocks against a woman's true freedom and equality. As long as she must forever bear and care for the result of conception so that her body, mind and spirit are bound by a *biological determinism,* she cannot know true liberty.

    (See *Christianity and Crisis* 32:292-295, January 8, 1973, p. 294.) To define "true liberty" in terms of total liberation from biological determinism is an angelicism worthy of Plotinus.

52. Plé, A., O.P., "Alert au traducianisme. Apropos de l'avortement", *Le Vie Spirituelle,* Supplement, 24:70, 1971.

53. See Theiner, J., *Die Entwiklung der Moraltheologie zur eigenstandigen Diziplin,* Regensburg, 1970; Haring, Bernard, *The Law of Christ,* 2 vols., de la theologie moral moderne", *Studia Moralia* I, Ancora, editor, Rome, 1962, pp. 87-120.

54. See the discussion of this in the distinguished Lutheran ethicist, Helmut Thielicke's "The Conflict Situation as Typical of Man's Ethical Relations to the World", *Theological Ethics,* Vol. I, Philadelphia: Fortress Press, 1966, pp. 482 ff.

55. The classical example of this is the difference between the Catholic casuistry of "mental

reservations" as a solution to truth-telling in a conflict situation, and Thielicke's solution which advises to "lie honestly" in such cases (see *ibid.,* "Compromise and the Limits of Truthfulness", pp. 520-566. A study of the two approaches shows that in fact they arrive at very much the same practical conclusions!)

56. Recently reasserted as follows: "The gravity of the problem comes from the fact that in certain cases, perhaps in quite a considerable number of cases, by denying abortion one endangers important values to which it is normal to attach great weight, and which may sometimes even seem to have priority. We do not deny these very great difficulties. It may be a serious question of health, sometimes of life or death, for the mother; it may be the importance attributed in different classes of society to considerations of honor or dishonor, of loss of social standing, and so forth. We proclaim only that none of these reasons can ever objectively confer the right to dispose of another's life, even when that life is only beginning." *Declaration on Procured Abortion,* Sacred Congregation for the Doctrine of the Faith, November 18, 1974.

57. See, for example, *Absolutes in Moral Theology,* Curran, Charles, editor, Washington: Corpus Books, 1968, and McCormick, Richard A., S.J., *Ambiguity in Moral Choice,* the 1973 Pere Marquette Theology Lecture, Marquette University, Milwaukee for a discussion of developments in Catholic theology aiming at a more adequate handling of conflict situations. Several approaches have been put forward, some, like Curran's "theology of compromise" coming very close to classical Protestant positions; others, like McCormick's, are closer to the casuistic tradition.

58. Curran, Charles, "Abortion: Its Legal and Moral Aspects in Catholic Theology", *New Perspectives in Moral Theology,* Notre Dame: Fides, 1974, pp. 163-68. Also see Donceel, Joseph, S.J., "Immediate Animation and Delayed Hominization", *Theological Studies* 31:106-124 for his attempt to revive the theory of "delayed animation". (But see Appendix I for a critique of the Theory of Delayed Hominization.)

59. Wasmer, Thomas A., S.J., "Contemporary Attitudes of the Roman Catholic Church Toward Abortion", *Journal of Religion and Health* 7:311-23, October, 1968; and Dedek, John, *Human Life: Some Moral Issues,* New York: Sheed and Ward, 1972, pp. 59 ff.

60. Gustafson, James M., "A Protestant Ethical Approach", *The Morality of Abortion: Legal and Historical Perspectives,* Noonan, John T., Jr., editor, Cambridge, Massachusetts: Harvard University Press, 1970, pp. 101-122; and *Theology and Christian Ethics,* Philadelphia: United Church Press, 1974; also, Fackre, Gabriel, "The Ethics of Abortion in Theological Perspective", *Andover-Newton Quarterly* 13:222-226, January, 1973; Ramsey's work mentioned in note 41 above.

5

Core Ethical Issues in Fetal Experimentation

The preceding chapters have reviewed the apparent widespread consensus that the human fetus is endowed with a basic human dignity worthy of protection by the adult community. However, in order to facilitate agreement on the kind and degree of protection that should be offered the fetus, the present chapter discusses several core ethical issues that are consequent upon human fetal dignity of the fetus. Accordingly, the ethical issues to be presented here will be raised in three successive reflections: a) The Human Fetus and the Principle of Equality, b) Fetal Experimentation and Community Ethical Values, and c) Implications of Ethically Regulated Fetal Experimentation for Scientific Progress.

The Human Fetus and the Principle of Equality

The three previous parts of this study have presented converging argumentation establishing the rights of the human fetus to the concern, care and protection of the adult community. Chapter II argued from the standpoint of the commitment of a civilized community to its weakest and least influential members. Chapter III argued from the personalist community and the developing personhood of the fetus. Chapter IV argued from Biblical teaching and the tradition of the Church that the I-Thou relation of God with human persons antecedes both birth and infancy.

These converging lines of reasoning indicate forcefully the need for serious ethical reflection about the implications of the human dignity of the fetuses. They indicate the error of those who would consider the human fetus merely as an "object" or as having a *"potential* human life." If such were the case, all forms of fetal research could easily be justified in much the same way as animal research. No serious objection could then be lodged against possible exploitation of human fetal life since fetuses would have no human dignity and such research would offer great hope of scientific progress in overcoming disease, deformity and spontaneous abortion.

However, the reasoning already presented indicates that fetuses must at least be considered "human subjects" of biomedical research. Thus fetal experimentation most appropriately was considered by the National Commission for the Protection of *Human Subjects* of Biomedical and Behavioral Research (Emphasis added).

The above reasoning has scientific, philosophical and theological foundations. Scientifically, the science of biology must classify the human fetus as a "living human being." A remark of Dr. André Hellegers can serve as a concise summary and reminder of the argument developed in Chapter III: "The fetus is an undoubted biological human being in the medical sense. It is human because it falls in the biological category of the human rather than in that of cats, rats or elephants. It is a being because it is there."[1]

Hellegers went on in the same discussion to indicate that value judgments are necessitated whenever the subject is a biological human being:

> In the abortion debate the physician can only state his own perceptions on value judgments about undoubted biological human life. For myself I have no difficulty in stating them simply. I believe that I can either look at differences between human beings and find therein a warranty for their destruction, or I can look at the likenesses and find in them a warranty for protection. I would like to be recorded among the protectors.[2]

The reluctance of scientists to make these value judgments in the name of science emphasizes the need for a broad consensus of the human community to make such judgments. Philosophy and theology assist in that regard. As indicated above in Chapter II the civilized human community can reason to a consensus on protecting the fetus as a human subject simply because the fetus is already a distinct, even if not independent, member of the political community. The personalist community can reach this consensus by reflecting on the continuity of the personhood process initiated at conception. Even the philosophical theory of delayed hominization recognizes the humanity of the fetus-subject from conception.[3] Finally, in Chapter IV, the basis was presented for a consensus of the Judaeo-Christian community on the dignity of the fetus as a human subject because of the unique relationship of human beings to the Creator.

Essential to all these reflections is the backward look from the natal moment of newborn human infants. The neonatal infant is clearly accepted as a human subject and in looking backward toward conception no satisfactory point of emergence of the human subject can be found subsequent to conception itself.

If a consensus were reached on considering human fetuses as "human subjects" does this mean that all fetuses would enjoy moral equality with all other members of the human species? As mentioned above in Chapter III, the principle of the moral equality of human beings demands a uniquely human, quantitatively immeasurable and qualitatively equal value of *all* human beings. It dictates humanitarian concern for the least privileged and most helpless members of the species. When understood as a normative principle it prescinds from such functional human activities as thinking, conscious reflection and free choice. The fetus has been identified as a member of the human species despite its inability to perform these functional human activities. Therefore moral equality may legitimately be predicated of three different human subjects: one who exercises the use of reason, one who has lost its exercise through mental dysfunction, and one (a fetus) who has not yet begun to exercise the use of reason. This means that from conception onwards, all human fetuses may claim moral equality with all other living human beings.

The assertion of this claim could well be coupled in life conflict situations with standard priorities for more developed human individuals. Many serious ethicists would countenance abortion to save the life of a mother without considering this a denial of the moral equality of mother and fetus. However, the widespread practice of abortion on request *does* in fact compromise the principle of moral equality since human fetuses are sacrificed in favor of lesser human values than the life of the mother, such as her physical comfort, economic or mental well-being, or her desired freedom from maternal responsibility.

As outlined above in Chapter IV, some contemporary Christian theologians have advanced a position which recognizes the fetus as a human subject but which suggests a developing scale of comparative human value as the fetus passes through gestation to birth. This position would legitimize abortion in other situations than life conflict situations. It would deny that human fetuses participate fully in moral equality with other human subjects. It would imply that some transition point other than conception must occur, whether at birth or at some indefinable point prior to, or even at some point following birth when the human fetus achieves fully human value. This study has failed to substantiate such a transition other than conception for the beginning of fully human value although the theory of delayed hominization would claim to find such a point early in gestation.

However, even the proponents of delayed hominization and of the theology cited above recognizes that the fetus is a human *subject* from conception. This offers an important consideration for the discussion of fetal experimentation. For even if the developing human fetuses do not enjoy full moral equality with other human beings, they do enjoy moral equality with other fetuses at the same stage of development. In other words, the admission that fetuses are human subjects indicates that they do enjoy in *some* degree, at least, the unique and indefinable kind of existence which cannot logically be curtailed by a discriminatory selection from other fetuses of their class who have the same claim on life that they have.

Logically, then, members of the class of human fetuses enjoy moral equality with others of their class. Discriminatory application of any selection process among comparable fetuses will violate that moral equality. For example, healthier fetuses do not have *more* developing humanness than the less healthy ones. Those with a more satisfactory genetic heritage do not have *more* developing humanness than those, for example, with a genetic predisposition for sickle cell anemia. Discrimination against "defective" fetuses would thus represent a prejudicial selection of human subjects in violation of their moral equality with each other. Those, then, who countenance abortion for such genetic reasons have overlooked this moral equality among human fetuses in addition to their bypassing of the moral equality of fetuses with other human subjects. If the quality of being human is possessed equally by all fetuses of the same stage of development despite variations in secondary characteristics, these latter characteristics should not be accepted for discriminatory policies at the cost of injustice and inhumanity. Most humanists would reject such a selection process among more developed human subjects; there is no compelling reason to excuse it among less developed human subjects like fetuses.

Obviously these considerations bear very directly on the issue of fetal experimentation, which can now be faced directly.

Fetal Experimentation and Community Ethical Values

The National Commission for the Protection of Human Subjects of Biomedical and Behavioral Research defined therapeutic research as "research designed to improve the health condition of the research subject by prophylactic, diagnostic or treatment methods that depart from standard medical practice but hold out a reasonable expectation of success."[4] Its definition of non-therapeutic research was purely negative: "research not designed to improve the health condition of the research subject by prophylactic, diagnostic or treatment methods."[5] Obviously the positive element implicit in responsible non-therapeutic research which should be spelled out explicitly - as indicated previously (pp. 12-13) - is the expected benefit to other human beings by the expected useful expansion of medical knowledge.

The Fetus and Informed Consent

Therapeutic experimentation offers few ethical problems if it is done responsibly and the expected benefit outweighs the risk to the human subject. In the case of a child or a fetus, the necessary consent for such therapy can be granted by a proxy, normally, a parent or legal guardian, since it may safely be presumed that the child or fetus would wish the benefit of therapeutic experimentation if he or she were able to give informed and free consent. A complete outline of ethical principles for human experimentation was presented in the Nuremburg Code after the Nazi excesses were uncovered.[6] The first of the ten points of this famous Code clearly designated the requisite qualities of voluntary consent, while the remaining points were addressed to other important considerations. Recently, The Department of Health, Education and Welfare has published its policy regarding the participation of *adult* human subjects in experimentation and included the requisite components of informed consent. The basic notions are that the patient be informed of the possible risks and expected benefits, and that he be able to make a decision free of any coercion and that he is at liberty to discontinue participation.[7]

However, non-therapeutic experimentation poses new ethical problems. It would seem that traditional ethical systems which oppose suicide would also oppose free consent by adults to experimentation that would be equivalently suicidal despite altruistic motivation for future scientific benefits.

Non-therapeutic experimentation on children and fetuses poses special problems concerning consent and the evaluation of risk. Paul Ramsey has pointed out the lack of careful limitations on proxy consent for non-therapeutic experimentation with children in both the Declaration of Helsinki's *Recommendations Guiding Doctors in Clinical Research* and the A.M.A.'s *Ethical Guidelines for Clinical Investigation.*[8] Ramsey argues that the altruism of an adult in submitting to non-therapeutic research involving risk to himself may not be attributed to a child or fetus as if the adult giving consent had absolute dominion over the child or fetus.[9] William May has argued in support of Ramsey's position which forbids all forms of non-therapeutic experimentation of children and fetuses.[10]

However, the positions of Ramsey and May are considered overly rigid by Richard McCormick.[11] Ramsey and May argue that the child is not a moral agent and hence can never be presumed to function as a volunteer for non-therapeutic research. But McCormick argues that even a child can be the subject of a moral obligation to consent to non-therapeutic research which offers him no discernible risk of harm and which offers significant benefit to the community. McCormick argues that a child, or a fetus, belongs to the human community and may be expected to render such a minimal service to the community at no significant cost to himself. Stephen Toulmin slightly reformulated McCormick's position in his study for the National Commission to avoid the seeming imputation of a moral action to the child or fetus by suggesting that non-therapeutic experimentation without discernible risk can be consented to in behalf of a child or fetus, since *if he were a moral agent,* he could not reasonably object.[12]

The authors of this study are persuaded that both secular and Christian ethical humanism can accept the position of McCormick. They feel it can be safely granted that proxy consent may be given for non-therapeutic research in cases where, in McCormick's words, "there is no discernible risk or undue discomfort," (yet, where there is genuine hope for general benefit).[13] Likely examples of such permissible non-therapeutic research would be: simple observation in a non-invasive manner, the use of amniotic fluid initially obtained for therapeutic reasons for additional experiments, and the use of information for therapeutically indicated ultrasound studies for research unrelated to that particular fetus.

The Factor of Risk

These fairly evident examples of experimentation without discernible risk lead to the important issue of "risk" in the cases of human fetuses. The notion of "risk" for given fetuses is open either to a generalized or an individualized kind of estimate. In the generalized interpretation, risk will be calculated from the amount of possible harm in the immediate or remote future to *any* fetus of comparable age and development subjected to the procedure contemplated. In the individualized interpretation, risk will be calculated from the amount of possible harm to this *particular* fetus which may be marked for abortion or which may have already been aborted, with little prospect for any remote future existence and future harm. "Risk" of harm becomes rather inconsequential in this latter case, so that practically unrestricted experimentation could be justified. However, it seems that the individualized interpretation of risk clearly violates the principle of the equality of all fetuses at a given stage of development as outlined in an earlier part of this chapter.

In other words, any attempt to make particular applications of the "risk" concept to fetuses destined for abortion or those already deliberately aborted constitutes unfair discrimination against them. Proxy consent for experimentation on these fetuses which are not scheduled for abortion exploits the individual situation of those fetuses marked for abortion. In effect, it says, "You have been condemned to die, therefore, the community will take advantage of your precarious situation and will utilize your research potential."

The implication of this discrimination by an individualized interpretation of "risk" is that some members of the research community will extrapolate consent for abortion into consent for experimentation. The persuasive appeal of merging these two consents into one was well expressed by Willard Gaylin and Marc Lappé in an article entitled "Fetal Politics: The Debate on Experimenting with the Unborn":

> In abortion, we condone procedures which subject the fetus to dismemberment, salt-induced osmotic shock, or surgical extirpation. No experimentation so far imagined would do the same. If society can condone abortion procedures which subject the live fetus to these unimaginable acts of violence, how can it balk at giving a mother an aspirin prior to those procedures in order to determine if the drug crosses the placenta with the hope that the knowledge thereby gained will prevent damage to future wanted babies?[14]

But Paul Ramsey has pointed out the pattern of the ethical illogicality of this position which presumes that one evil can justify another. He notes that the community-benefit argumentation constitutes a "salvation" rationalization.[15] The "hope that the knowledge thereby gained will prevent damage to future wanted babies" is considered a "saving grace" but one evil cannot be "saved" by another. Researchers who extend a proxy consent for abortion into a proxy consent for experimentation which, of itself, offers significant risk to fetuses of a comparable development must recognize that they are party to a *new* indignity and a *new* form of discrimination projected on the fetus. Just as two wrongs do not make a right, two successive misuses of proxy consent do not make a right use of consent.

For fetuses who are accepted as having full moral equality with other human beings abortion clearly constitutes an act of injustice - except possibly in those cases where the life of the mother is at stake. Those who judge the fetus not to have full moral equality with other human beings, will justify an abortion by a pregnant mother on the grounds that some personal human good outweighs the values of this human subject. The mother also may attempt to justify her decision by arguing that *this* present fetus conflicts with *her* specific human good. However, should the research community use this fetus for the hoped-for benefit of future fetuses, it still has no title whatsoever to exploit *this* fetus: this fetus is not, in any sense, in conflict with any human goods of the community whatsoever. The community may have tolerated the mother's choice, but this does not establish ethical grounds for experimentation upon this fetus.

Normally, scientific researchers may not use arbitrary discrimination or accidental availability in selecting research subjects. In the case of adults the necessity of free and informed consent limits non-therapeutic research to actual volunteers. In the case of children, researchers would not usually expect to exploit research subjects with a limited longevity expectation unless their research was therapeutic or offered no discernible risk. The fact that pregnant mothers choose abortion and decide upon limited longevity for their fetuses constitutes accidental availability, but does not justify the research community in pursuing this discriminatory selection of human subjects for non-therapeutic experimentation. If the research community attempts to exploit the sampling of fetuses provided by abortion on the grounds that they possess less than full human dignity, it will go beyond *Roe v. Wade*, which tolerated a woman's "right" to an abortion but did not give the community any "right" to extend further the abortion consent.

The rationale of this extension has already been referred to in the "salvation" imagery of Gaylin and Lappé, who write that "it (fetal research) endows the process of abortion with human values it will not otherwise have."[16] This line of reasoning invokes the classical cost/benefit analysis and the calculations of utilitarian ethics. But even so, it involves the subordination of individuals to community benefit in a way that civilized communities have come to reject in favor of the rights of human members. No one would select a sample of the infant population, for instance, for an activity with grave risks on the grounds of community benefit. Even in a utilitarian ethic, this would be excluded because it would not be useful for the stability and well-being of the community in the long range.

Some may argue that the abortion decision of individual mothers has already made available a sample of human subjects, and non-therapeutic experimentation will simply reap positive community benefits from their actions. But this overlooks the fact that non-therapeutic research adds to the process of abortion a new initiative in the experimental procedure. Non-therapeutic research with discernible risk ethically cannot be imposed on condemned criminals in modern society or on dying children; by the same reasoning it should not be imposed on aborted fetuses or fetuses marked for abortion.

In the light of this study it would seem that the only satisfactory justification for the discriminatory treatment of fetuses-to-be-aborted or of those already aborted is based on the assumption that such fetuses are not "human subjects" at all. Logically consistent as such a justification may be, it has been rejected by the considerations above in Chapters II, III and IV. Because of the converging argumentation this rejection is not based exclusively on Christian or Catholic beliefs, even though they do articulate the human status of the fetus very clearly. On the other hand, this conclusion should be accepted by those ethicists of a utilitarian bent who concede that fetuses are "human subjects." They do not ordinarily use the utilitarian principle of the greatest good for the greatest number to justify torturing human subjects. A serious form of massive dehumanization was introduced by use of the utilitarian principle to justify the eugenicist policies of National Socialism in Germany.

Logically the compromise of the equal dignity of fetuses for consequential benefits to the community at large cannot be clearly distinguished from compromising under similar circumstances the equal dignity of other classes in society, e.g., infants, adolescents, or senior citizens. Fetuses are morally equal at least to others of their comparable age and development, if not to all human beings, as long as they are human subjects in the first place. Discrimination against fetuses *accidentally* chosen for abortion by maternal decision would be comparable to discrimination against senior citizens *accidentally* chosen for active euthanasia by governmental edict. One may argue that senior citizens have greater human dignity than fetuses (as discussed above) but one may not deny the comparable fact of discrimination and unjustified exploitation of the individuals selected.

To allow such discrimination to capitalize on women's abortion decisions is to admit that developing human subjects, whatever the occasions which make them available, can be sacrificed to the community's scientific progress and the well-being of future individuals. This study indicates that this sacrifice is both unchristian and inhuman in terms of ethical judgment.

Concluding Propositions

1. The human fetus is not mere tissue or animal life or a *potential* human person (but is a potential adult person).
2. The human fetus is a human subject from conception with an active potential for developing as a person and therefore shares moral equality at least with other human fetuses in comparable stages of development, if not with all other human beings.
3. The factual situation of an abortion having taken place or being contemplated must not be presumed to deprive the fetus of inherent human dignity any more than a death sentence accomplishes this with a condemned criminal.
4. Regardless of the moral evaluation of the abortion decision, an independent judgment must be made of the rightness or wrongness of unrestricted non-therapeutic fetal experimentation. The imminent death decreed by abortion could only justify the latter if propositions 1) and 2) above were overthrown.
5. Submitting fetuses destined for abortion, or already aborted, to risks which would be significant for fetuses destined to be carried to term constitutes a discriminatory practice in the light of 2) above.
6. The discriminatory practice in using fetuses as subjects who have been selected for abortion for non-therapeutic experimentation amounts to sacrificing fetal human dignity for the sake of scientific progress—an unacceptable procedure analogous to sacrificing the dignity of an infant or a senior citizen to scientific progress.
7. Such a sacrifice cannot be justified on utilitarian grounds without either denying that fetuses are human subjects (1) and (2) above or opening a wedge whereby other selected human subjects can be exploited for community purposes.

Ethical Constraints and Fetal Experimentation: Implications for Scientific Progress

The ethical reasoning presented above by no means eliminates all fetal experimentation and research progress. The major source of scientific progress in fetology and pre-natal studies until very recently came primarily from therapeutic experimentation and non-invasive observational techniques which present no ethical problems. Widespread practice of newly-legalized induced abortion has only recently offered possibilities of controlled research without therapeutic benefit on fetuses both *in utero,* during abortion, and alive *ex utero.* The ethical implications of these new possibilities precipitated this lengthy study.

As indicated, the above ethical argumentation would not permit non-therapeutic experimentation which offers significant risk to human fetuses when the risk is interpreted in a generalized rather than in an individualized sense. It would not permit, therefore, experiments on fetuses about to be aborted, or already aborted and possibly viable, if these experiments offered significant risk to comparable fetuses intended to be brought to term. In the case of clearly living but possibly viable fetuses surviving outside the womb, all therapeutic procedures could still be employed even with minimal hope of success. But non-therapeutic procedures which offered significant risk to the future well-being of such fetuses, should they survive, would be prohibited.

The authors of this study are unable to offer any reliable calculation of the differing rates of scientific progress in fetology if these norms were to be followed, as opposed to the presumed larger and faster rate of scientific progress if less restrictive norms permitting non-therapeutic fetal experimentation were applied.[17] Progress will surely not halt in the former case and it would seem likely even to continue to accelerate simply because of the "snowball effect" of research itself and of the current increased availability of human fetuses for non-therapeutic minimal risk experimentation. Therefore the incalculable, but presumably greater rate of progress with less limited experimentation should be foregone so as to avoid the incalculable but presumably greater rate of moral deterioration and "brutalization" which would likewise follow. This latter presumption, at least, has in its favor the experience of Nazi Germany and of many other instances in human history where respect for individual rights has gradually been blunted by the acceptance of dehumanizing practices.

In conclusion, even if significant scientific benefits exclusively available through unrestricted fetal experimentation could be documented, they would not justify it any more than comparable experimentation could be justified on human infants. This means that a policy based on the ethical reasoning outlined above offers the wisest course for the human community and a refusal to compromise must be made now, if even more difficult decisions are to be forestalled in the future.

Summary

Consideration of the core ethical issues in fetal experimentation leads to the conclusion that the rightness or wrongness of unrestricted non-therapeutic fetal experimentation must be made independently of the moral evaluation of abortion. Because the fetus is not a *potential* human person (albeit the fetus is a potential human *adult*) but is a human subject from conception, he shares moral equality with other human fetuses and thus may not be discriminated against within his own class. There is no convincing evidence that respect for the moral equality of fetuses and their human dignity would significantly impair medical progress. The *rate* of advance may be somewhat reduced, but to increase its pace at the cost of injustice to individual fetuses is not justifiable.

CHAPTER V Footnotes

1. "The Beginnings of Personhood: Medical Considerations", *The Perkins Journal of Theology,* Fall 1973, Vol. 27, No. 1, p. 14.
2. *Ibid.,*
3. For instance, Joseph Donceel, S.J. wrote in a recent article: "Science has demonstrated that the embryo is a human organism from the beginning, that it is, physiologically speaking, a human being." See "Why Is Abortion Wrong?" *America,* August 16, 1975, Vol. 133, No. 4, p. 66.
4. "Toward a Policy on Fetal Research", *Origins,* June 12, 1975, Vol. 5, No. 3, p. 35. See also *Federal Register,* August 8, 1975.
5. *Ibid.,* p. 35.
6. See Beecher, Henry K., *Research and the Individual,* Boston: Little, Brown and Co., 1970, Appendix A, pp. 227-229.
7. *Federal Register* 39 (105): 18917, May 30, 1974. "(c) "Informed consent" means the knowing consent of an individual or his legally authorized representative, so situated as to be able to exercise free power of choice without undue inducement or any element of force, fraud, deceit, duress, or other form of constraint or coercion. The basic elements of information necessary to such consent include:
   (1) A fair explanation of the procedures to be followed, and their purposes, including identification of any procedures which are experimental;
   (2) A description of any attendant discomforts and risks reasonably to be expected;
   (3) A description of any benefits reasonably to be expected;
   (4) A disclosure of any appropriate alternative procedures that might be advantageous for the subject;
   (5) An offer to answer any inquiries concerning the procedures; and
   (6) An instruction that the person is free to withdraw his consent and to discontinue participation in the project or activity at any time without prejudice to the subject."
8. *Patient as Person,* New Haven, Connecticut: Yale University Press, 1970, p. 19.
9. *Op. cit.* Also Ramsey, Paul, *The Ethics of Fetal Research,* New Haven, Connecticut: Yale University Press, 1975.
10. "Experimenting on Human Subjects", *Linacre Quarterly,* November, 1974, Vol. 41, No. 4, pp. 238-252.
11. "Fetal Research, Morality , and Public Policy", *Hastings Center Report,* June, 1975, Vol. 5, No. 3, p. 27. See also McCormick, Richard, "Proxy Consent in the Experimentation Situation", *Perspectives in Biology and Medicine,* 18, 1974, pp. 2-20.
12. "Exploring the Moderate Consensus", *Hastings Center Report,* June, 1975, Vol. 5, No. 3, p. 34.
13. McCormick, *op. cit.,* as in Note 10. above.
14. "Fetal Politics", *Atlantic,* May, 1975, Vol. 235, pp. 66-71; see p. 66.
15. Ramsey, *The Ethics of Fetal Research,* pp. 42-44.
16. *Op. cit.,* p. 71.
17. While instances can be cited of progress made through use of non-therapeutic fetal experimentation which offered significant risk to the fetus, it is still difficult to estimate when or if such achievements might have been made by the kinds of experimentation considered ethically acceptable here. It is likewise impossible to estimate reliably what future achievements would be made with unrestricted fetal non-therapeutic experimentation. We note with sympathy and appreciation the comment of David Louisell: "Even if I were to approach my task as a commissioner from a utilitarian viewpoint only, I would have to say that on the record here I am not convinced that an adequate showing has been made of the necessity for non-therapeutic fetal experimentation in the scientific or social interest." See "A Breach of our Moral Tradition," *Origins,* June 12, 1975, Vol. 5, No. 3, p. 44.

6

Federal Regulation of Fetal Experimentation

In July, 1974, Congress passed the National Research Act, which imposed a temporary moratorium on research on fetuses either before or after induced abortion if carried out or financed by the Department of Health, Education and Welfare (DHEW). The Act also created the National Commission for the Protection of Human Subjects of Biomedical and Behavioral Research to study the legal, ethical, and medical aspects of scientific research on human subjects.[1] This last chapter of the study will consist first of an evaluation of the recommendations put forward by the Commission. Secondly, after evaluating these recommendations, the relevant federal regulations will be cited and discussed. A third major section concludes this chapter with an outline of the essential elements for a more satisfactory set of alternative regulations.

Recommendations of the National Commission - An Evaluation*

The first task assigned to the National Commission for the Protection of Human Subjects of Biomedical and Behavioral Research was extremely difficult. The Commission was asked to explore fetal experimentation, an uncommonly controversial topic, and to submit recommendations concerning such experimentation to the Secretary of DHEW. That study required that the demands, interests, and necessities of a pluralistic society, as well as the dignity of human subjects and the needs of scientific progress, be considered. On May 21, 1975, the Commission submitted its recommendations to Secretary Caspar W. Weinberger. In August, Weinberger lifted the year-long ban on fetal research and simultaneously

*The first part of this chapter has appeared in a slightly modified form in *Hospital Progress*, September, 1975, and is included here with the permission of the publisher.

issued regulations which are generally consistent with the Commission's recommendations. The regulations were published in the *Federal Register* of August 8, 1975.[2]

Given the difficulty of its task, the brief time allotted for formulating norms, and the novelty of the assignment, the Commission should be commended for its serious and open-minded work. Moreover, it deserves commendation for its exploratory method: an initial statement of the principles it intended to use followed by the application of these principles. However, as will be shown in the subsequent analysis, the Commission failed to apply these principles consistently when formulating its recommendations. As a consequence, certain of the federal regulations, consistent with the recommendations, endanger the thrust of modern humane tradition by potentially allowing harmful nontherapeutic research on nonconsenting human subjects.

This portion of our study is directed toward both the recommendations of the Commission which are the basis for the new federal regulations on fetal experimentation, and on the commentary prepared by the Commission, which is the key to their interpretation. The text of the Commission's report, which consists of an introductory commentary of guiding principles in addition to the recommendations themselves, may be found in the issue of the *Federal Register* mentioned above, or in *ORIGINS,* June 12, 1975, in which an unabridged version of the recommendations are published. Quotations taken from the Commission's commentary are referred to by letter and number

The National Commission's Ethical Principles for Medical Research

The Commission states: Among the general principles for research on human subjects to be valid and binding are:

1. "To avoid harm whenever possible, or at least to minimize harm";
2. "To provide for fair treatment by avoiding discrimination among members of the same class" (referred to as the principle of equality, (C.3);
3. "To respect the integrity of human subjects by requiring informed consent," and
4. "To respect the human character of the fetus" (B).

Later, when discussing the matter of risk and consent, the Commission lists a fifth principle: "The Commission affirms as a general principle that manifest risks imposed on nonconsenting subjects cannot be tolerated. Therefore, the Commission concludes that only minimal risk can be accepted as permissible for nonconsenting subjects in nontherapeutic research" (C.3).

In addition to these five principles, the Commission states certain general requirements as being necessary for ethical research upon fetuses. These would be ascertained in the review process which must precede approval of any research project. These general requirements are:

1. "Appropriate prior investigations using animal models and non-

pregnant humans must have been completed.

2. The knowledge to be gained must be important and obtainable by no reasonable alternative means.

3. Risks and benefits to both the mother and the fetus must have been fully evaluated and described.

4. Informed consent must be sought and granted under proper conditions.

5. Subjects must be selected so that risks and benefits will not fall inequitably among economic, racial, ethnic, and social classes." (B)

Each of these principles is valid, and each protects and fosters human dignity. If they had been applied consistently in accord with the express intention of the Commission to treat the fetus as "a human subject," then a humane and acceptable set of recommendations would more likely have been formulated. However, they were not applied consistently, one reason for which may have been insufficient time. The Commission stated that it had been "placed under severe limitation of time by its Congressional mandate. As a result, these considerations on research involving fetuses have necessarily been developed prior to the Commission's larger task of studying the nature of research, the basic ethical principles which should guide it, the problem of informed consent and the review process" (VIII).

Hence, the Commission admitted that it "has not yet studied the issues surrounding informed consent for nontherapeutic research" (VII, C). Yet it proceeded to approve recommendations, which, in order to be just and humane, theoretically require a clear notion of the principle of informed consent as well as the import of its corollary, that "manifest risks imposed upon nonconsenting adults cannot be tolerated."

That the Commission should have completed its consideration of consent before formulating recommendations would have been more important than meeting the Congressional deadline. The principle of informed consent is, after all, a primary one in regard to human research. The ramifications of compromising it for the purpose of potentially harmful experimentation are far-reaching. Our civilization is based upon respect for individual dignity and equality; one of its highest ideals is the protection of the weak and infirm from harm. It professes that the individual does not exist for the state and cannot be sacrificed unwillingly for the public welfare.

If the principles of informed consent are not followed faithfully and consistently, these values are seriously endangered. It would seem that in several of the recommendations to be discussed below, the Commission failed to establish sufficient safeguards in reference to the principle of consent and the limitation to only minimal or no risk.

Recommendations Concerning Therapeutic Research

The Commission's first two recommendations concern therapeutic research:

1. Therapeutic research directed toward the fetus may be conducted or supported, and should be encouraged, by the Secretary, DHEW, provided such research (a) conforms to appropriate medical standards; (b) has received the informed consent of the mother, the father not dissenting; and (c) has been approved by existing review procedures with adequate provision for the monitoring of the consent process. (Adopted unanimously.)
2. Therapeutic research directed toward the pregnant woman may be conducted or supported, and should be encouraged, by the Secretary, DHEW, provided such research (a) has been evaluated for possible impact on the fetus; (b) will place the fetus at risk to the minimum extent consistent with meeting the health needs of the pregnant woman; (c) has been approved by existing review procedures with adequate provision for the monitoring of the consent process; and (d) the pregnant woman has given her informed consent. (Adopted unanimously.)

The Commission generally concludes "that therapeutic research directed toward the health condition of either the fetus or the pregnant woman is, in principle, ethical. Such research benefits not only the individual woman or fetus, but also women and fetuses as a class, and should therefore be encouraged actively" (C,2). The first recommendation is adequate, but the second gives cause for concern, the reason being that research directed primarily toward the pregnant woman in many cases will affect the fetus as well, and it is important that the rights of the fetus also be clearly protected. Recognizing that "the therapeutic research directed toward the pregnant woman may expose the fetus to risk for the benefit of another subject," the Commission makes some effort to protect the fetus by stating that the research upon a pregnant woman may be supported, provided that such research will "put the fetus at minimum risk consistent with the provision of health care for the woman." But the actual protection afforded the fetus is extremely tenuous because the Commission recognizes "the woman's priority regarding her own health care " (VII, C,2). This latter phrase would allow research that would injure or even destroy the fetus if it were "consistent with the health needs of the mother." If the term "health of the mother" is interpreted as it was in the Supreme Court decision regarding abortion, (and there is no reason to think that this precedent will not be followed), then any research which treats a pregnant woman for emotional or psychological difficulty, as well as for physiological maladies, could justify research endangering the fetus. In such cases, the fetus would not be treated as a "human subject in scientific research" as the Commission avowed it should. Rather, in spite of some palliative language, the fetus would be treated as an object to be discarded if the "health needs of the pregnant woman" should warrant it.

Acknowledging the Supreme Court decision which subordinated the fetus' right to life and the right to due process to the woman's right to privacy, *(Roe v. Wade, Doe v. Bolton),* the Commission might have felt unable to give greater recognition to the fetus' right to be considered a human subject. If the Supreme Court decisions are to be used as the sole standard for the formulation of fetal experimentation norms, then how can these norms possibly be humane if, according to these decisions, the fetus has no right to be treated as a human subject, no right to life, and no right to human dignity? Rightful consideration would more likely be given to the fetus if the clause "consistent with meeting the health needs of the pregnant woman" were eliminated, and the woman's health did not automatically receive priority. In this way, the rights of the fetus and those of the woman would be balanced one against the other and a more equitable protection realized. Even though, under the guise of the right to privacy, the Supreme Court has denied the human fetus equal protection of the law, the Commission should not have made the same denial in the name of therapeutic research. As David Louisell, a member of the Commission who filed a dissenting opinion, stated when discussing another recommendation offered by the Commission: "While we must abide the Court's mandate in a particular case on the issues actually decided even though the decision is wrong and in fact only an exercise of 'raw judicial power' (White, J., dissenting in *Roe* and *Doe*), this does not mean we should extend an erroneous rationale to other situations."[3]

Recommendations Concerning Non-Therapeutic Research

Research directed toward the pregnant woman: The third through the seventh recommendations address nontherapeutic research: the third is concerned primarily with the pregnant woman; the others, with the fetus at various stages of development.

> 3. Nontherapeutic research directed toward the pregnant woman may be conducted or supported by the Secretary, DHEW, provided such research (a) has been evaluated for possible impact on the fetus; (b) will impose minimal or no risk to the well-being of the fetus; (c) has been approved by existing review procedures with adequate provision for the monitoring of the consent process; (d) special care has been taken to assure that the woman has been fully informed regarding possible impact on the fetus; and (e) the woman has given informed consent. (Adopted unanimously.)
> It is further provided that nontherapeutic research directed at the pregnant woman may be conducted or supported (f) only if the father has not objected, both where abortion is not at issue (adopted by a vote of 8 to 1) and where an abortion is anticipated (adopted by a vote of 5 to 4).

In recommendation No. 3, the Commission considers nontherapeutic research directed toward the pregnant woman. Once again, the key question is: Will the fetus be respected as a human subject? The Commission seems to recognize the right of the fetus to be protected, for it concludes in recommendation No. 3 that nontherapeutic research directed toward a pregnant woman should be funded only if the research "(a) has been evaluated for possible impact upon the well-being of the fetus; and (b) will impose minimal or no risk to the well-being of the fetus." However, the Commission also admits that "the term minimal risk involves a value judgment and acknowledges that medical opinion will differ in regard to what constitutes minimal risk" (VIII, C.3). The main factor causing differences of opinion about minimal risk appears to be whether or not the fetus will be aborted. The concept of minimal risk applied to the case of a fetus going to term would be different, according to some Commission members, from that one which will be aborted. Their thought, then, seems to be: if the fetus is going to be destroyed, then less care need be devoted to it.

The Commission states that in any research procedure, the "determination of acceptable minimal risk is a function of the review process." But the door is clearly open for those conducting the review process to apply more lenient norms for minimal risk in the case of fetuses to be aborted than for those who will be carried to term. According to the report, "There is a basic agreement among Commission members as to the validity of the equality principle. There is disagreement as to its application to individual fetuses and classes of fetuses" (VIII, C.3). It seems, however, that the absence of more definitive protection from harmful experimentation for the fetus-to-be-aborted amounts to a disavowal and contradiction of the equality principle, not merely a disagreement in regard to its application.

Indeed, to allow human subjects to be used for medical research experimentation simply because they will soon die, especially if the research were potentially harmful, is a departure from the recent medical tradition of Western civilization which lavishes so much care on the sick. If the Commission wished to grant the fetus its rights as a human subject, it should have refused to consider the possibility of any research which would allow the fetus to be treated differently simply because it would later be aborted. This would put "minimal risk" into proper context. The Commission considered this possibility and rejected it (VIII, C.3).

Research directed toward the fetus in utero:

4. Nontherapeutic research directed toward the fetus *in utero* (other than research in anticipation of, or during, abortion) may be conducted or supported by the Secretary, DHEW, provided (a) the purpose of such research is the development of important biomedical knowledge that cannot be obtained by alternative means; (b) investigation on pertinent animal models and nonpregnant humans has preceded such research; (c) minimal or no risk to the well-being of the fetus will be imposed by the research; (d) the research has been approved by existing review procedures with adequate provision for the monitoring of the consent process; (e) the informed consent of the mother has been obtained; and (f) the father has not objected to the research. (Adopted unanimously.)

The fourth recommendation concerns nontherapeutic research directed toward the fetus *in utero* when abortion is not anticipated. Were this well-stated recommendation applicable to all fetuses, including those to be aborted, then the Commission would have written norms completely in accord with its own principles and the medical tradition of Western civilization.

> 5. Nontherapeutic research directed toward the fetus in anticipation of abortion may be conducted or supported by the Secretary, DHEW, provided such research is carried out within the guidelines for all other nontherapeutic research directed toward the fetus *in utero.* Such research presenting special problems related to the interpretation or application of these guidelines may be conducted or supported by the Secretary, DHEW, provided such research has been approved by a national ethical review body." (Adopted by a vote of 8 to 1.)

The fifth recommendation considers the situation of nontherapeutic research directed toward the fetus in anticipation of abortion. This recommendation stipulates that research involving fetuses-to-be-aborted must conform to "the guidelines for all other nontherapeutic research directed toward the fetus *in utero.*" This recommendation is acceptable provided that application of the principle of "minimal risk" does not vary nor is more liberal in the case of a fetus-to-be-aborted. It seems that the recommendation would be safer if clarifying and limiting language were added.

After seemingly protecting the fetus-to-be-aborted from harmful research, the Commission provides for exceptional cases by inserting a clause which could destroy such protection. This clause states that:

> research presenting special problems related to the interpretation or application of these guidelines may be conducted or supported by the DHEW Secretary, provided that such research has been approved by a national ethical review body.

This statement may result in practices which contradict the previously enunciated principle of the Commission that "only minimal risk can be accepted as permissible for non-consenting subjects in nontherapeutic research" (C,3). As Louisell declares in his minority report, this clause should be omitted and in its place there should be a declaration substituted that "no research should be permitted on a fetus-to-be-aborted that would not be permitted on one to go to term."[4] The decision that a woman makes to have an abortion should not make it possible for a human fetus to be used in a manner contrary to its inherent human dignity, notwithstanding what personal, civic or research interests might be involved.

Research directed toward the premature, nonsurviving infant: The sixth recommendation concerns nontherapeutic research directed toward the fetus during the abortion procedure and the nonviable fetus *ex utero:*

> 6. Nontherapeutic research directed toward the fetus during the abortion procedure and nontherapeutic research directed toward the nonviable fetus *ex utero* may be conducted or supported by the Secretary, DHEW, provided (a) the purpose of such research is the development of important biomedical knowlege that cannot be obtained by alternative means; (b) investigation on pertinent animal models and nonpregnant humans (when appropriate) has preceded such research; (c) the research has been approved by existing review procedures with adequate provision for the monitoring of the consent process; and (e) the father has not objected to the research; and provided further that (f) the fetus is less than 20 weeks gestational age; (g) that no significant procedural changes are introduced into the abortion procedure in the interest of research alone; and (h) no intrusion into the fetus is made which alters the duration of life. Such research presenting special problems related to the interpretation or application of these guidelines may be conducted or supported by the Secretary, DHEW, provided such research has been approved by a national ethical review body. (Adopted by a vote of 8 to 1.)

It might be pointed out in passing that *"fetus ex utero"* is an infelicitous term because the living fetus outside the womb, whether it will survive or not, is usually referred to as a human infant, as Louisell notes in his dissenting opinion.[5] Indeed, it is so designated in the Commission's seventh recommendation. Does the mere alteration of a term to justify exposure of such a premature infant inhuman treatment?

By the establishment of two sets of guidelines for research and experimentation, one for fetuses that will be aborted, and another for those that will not be aborted, the Commission has violated its own principle of equality. The Commission maintains that "respect for the dignity of the fetus continues to be of paramount importance" and that it wishes "the fetus to be treated with the respect due to dying subjects" (C,4). While it appears to put these statements into practice by declaring that the dying fetus' life may not be extended or shortened by proposed research, it does not go far enough. Harmful experimentation short of altering the duration of life would then be allowed. If the dignity of the fetus as a dying subject is of "paramount importance," and if its integrity is a "central" issue (C,4), then all fetuses should be treated equally. Dying fetuses which result from elective abortions should not be treated as a distinct category.

The term "nonviable fetus ex utero" is used to designate a human subject that is alive, but which, according to the best medical evidence and judgment, will not survive, even with the aid of the best available life support technology. Traditionally, such a human subject has been called a premature infant. While it may not be possible to change the terminology used by the Commission and the DHEW, the use of this new term should not allow for this type of human subject to be treated as anything other than a living human being. Hence, the infant in question should receive the same respect and care as any other living human subject.

Hence, research and experimentation upon dying fetuses which would not be permitted on viable fetuses should be prohibited. The mere fact that a fetus is dying, no matter what the cause, does not constitute grounds for allowing harmful experimentation or for withdrawing the protection extended to other human subjects. Would experimentation with dying adults be permitted without their consent? If the dying are not able to give their consent, would harmful, nontherapeutic research be practiced upon them using only proxy consent? If the Commission declares that the fetus is to be treated as a "human subject in scientific research," and if it espouses consistent application of the principle of equality, then it must consider how other members of society are treated when research and experimentation are under consideration. It does not suffice for the Commission to say that the dying fetus cannot "be 'harmed' in the sense of "injured for life." If this recommendation is retained at all, it should stipulate that no additional harm be done to the dying fetus as a result of the research.

The same harmful "escape clause" at the end of the fifth recommendation is appended to the sixth as well. If this clause were eliminated from both recommendations, it would be more in accord with humanistic traditions and the principles espoused by the Commission. Both clauses would be revised to read that no research should be permitted on a fetus-to-be-aborted that would not be permitted on a fetus allowed to go to term.

Research directed toward the premature, possibly surviving infant: The seventh recommendation concerns research directed toward the possibly viable infant. It states:

> 7. Nontherapeutic research directed toward the possibly viable infant may be conducted or supported by the Secretary, DHEW, provided (a) the purpose of such research is the development of important biomedical knowledge that cannot be obtained by alternative means; (b) investigation on pertinent animal models and nonpregnant humans (when appropriate) has preceded such research; (c) no additional risk to the well-being of the infant will be imposed by the research; (d) the research has been approved by existing review procedures with adequate provision for the monitoring of the consent process; and (e) informed consent of either parent has been given and neither parent has objected. (Adopted unanimously.)

The rationale for this recommendation is that "there is, of course, a moral and legal obligation to attempt to save the life of a possibly viable infant" (C,4). Here, two considerations should be pointed out: First, defining a "possible viable infant" is indeed difficult, as is apparent in the very use of the word "possibly." What norms would be used to determine this "possible viability?" Certainly, new techniques such as *in vitro* fertilization and gestation will affect any norms adopted during the next few years. Hence, in response to its avowed principle "to attempt to save the life of a possibly viable infant," the Commission should make some reference in its review procedures to this possibility and the limiting effect it will have on future plans for research upon the fetus, which, at this time, might be considered nonviable.

Second, when discussing the harm that might come to the subject of research, the Commission uses the phrase "no additional risk to the well-being of the fetus will be imposed by the research," instead of "minimal or no risk to the well-being of the fetus will be imposed by research," which is the phrase used in the third and fourth recommendations. The question might be raised as to whether these phrases have the same meaning, and if so, would not the former phrases be more in keeping with the Commission's intention than the latter? The matter of proxy consent in nontherapeutic research is crucial to a humane approach to the matter of experimentation. Any language that clearly and definitively states this and which gives greater protection to the subject should be employed.

Other Recommendations

Review procedures: The eighth recommendation concerns review procedures, i.e., the procedures used to confirm the necessity for the research, and to insure that proper nonhuman research has preceded it, that risks and benefits have been fully evaluated, and that informed consent has been obtained. The recommendation follows:

> 8. Review procedures. Until the commission makes its recommendations regarding review and consent procedures, the review procedures mentioned above are to be those presently required by the DHEW. In addition, provision for monitoring the consent process shall be required in order to insure adequacy of the consent process and to prevent unfair discrimination in the selection of research subjects, for all categories of research mentioned above. A national ethical review, as required in recommendations 5 and 6, shall be carried out by an appropriate body designated by the Secretary, DHEW, until the establishment of the National Advisory Council for the Protection of Subjects of Biomedical and Behavioral Research. In order to facilitate public understanding and the presentation of public attitudes toward special problems reviewed by the national review body, appropriate provision should be made for public attendance and public participation in the national review process. (Adopted unanimously, one abstention.)

The first part of this recommendation concerns nontherapeutic research accompanied by minimal or no risk to the human subject. The

Commission concluded that the review procedures currently followed by DHEW are satisfactory (D). It added, however, that "the case is different . . . for nontherapeutic research directed toward a pregnant woman or a fetus if it involves more than minimal risk or would not be acceptable for application to an infant . . . In such cases, the Commission considers current review procedures insufficient" (D).

Hence, in the second paragraph of the eighth recommendation, the Commission calls for the DHEW Secretary to designate an appropriate body to address "special problems" envisioned in the fifth and sixth recommendations until the National Advisory Council for the Protection of Subjects of Biomedical and Behavioral Research is established. Once again, very strenuous objections to this provision must be raised because it allows for the possibility that nontherapeutic research which is harmful to the subject (more than minimal risk) could be carried on without the consent of the subject, or with only proxy consent, especially if such research would be of great "scientific and public value." No such value could justify nontherapeutic, harmful research upon nonconsenting human subjects. To compromise this principle is to seriously erode the civilized tradition of care and concern for the weak, the infirm, the young who cannot consent, and the adult who cannot resist coercion. The individual does not exist for society, although he may determine freely and knowingly at times to sacrifice himself for society.

Research on the dead fetus and fetal tissue: The ninth recommendation stipulates conditions for research on dead fetuses and fetal tissue:

> 9. Research on the dead fetus and fetal tissue. The commission recommends that use of the dead fetus, fetal tissue and fetal material for research purposes be permitted, consistent with local law, the Uniform Anatomical Gift Act and commonly held convictions about respect for the dead . (Adopted unanimously, one abstention.)

Thus, the recommendation states that local law, the Uniform Anatomical Gift Act, and commonly held convictions about respect for the dead will limit this research. What these "commonly held convictions about respect for the dead" are, however, the report does not clearly specify. Certainly, disputes will arise concerning the practical implementation of this recommendation, but accepted protocol for research upon dead adults could serve as a guide for conducting the review process. For example, some thought should be given to the matter of consent. Who will give the consent needed to release dead fetuses for research? Would the mother of an aborted fetus have relinquished this right by reason of her decision to have the fetus destroyed? Would the court be asked to grant permission? Or would it be presumed that dead fetuses, unlike dead adults, are public property and can be disposed of indiscriminately?[6]

Certainly, we must avoid situations which might result in illegal practices such as the trafficking in aborted fetuses in England.

Miscellaneous recommendations: The remaining recommendations are concerned with a number of disparate situations.

10. The design and conduct of a nontherapeutic research protocol should not determine recommendations by a physician regarding the advisability, timing or method of abortion. (Adopted by a vote of 6 to 2.)
11. Decisions made by a personal physician concerning the health care of a pregnant woman or fetus should not be compromised for research purposes, and when a physician of record is involved in a prospective research protocol, independent medical judgment on these issues is required.

    In such cases, review panels should assure that procedures for such independent medical judgment are adequate, and all conflict of interest or appearance thereof between appropriate health care and research objectives should be avoided. (Adopted unanimously.)
12. The commission recommends that research on abortion techniques continue as permitted by law and government regulation. (Adopted by a vote of 6 to 2.)
13. The commission recommends that attention be drawn to Section 214(d) of the National Research Act (PL 93-348) which provides that: "No individual shall be required to perform or assist in the performance of any part of a health service program or research activity funded in whole or in part by the Secretary of Health, Education, and Welfare if his performance or assistance in the performance of such part of such program or activity would be contrary to his religious beliefs or moral convictions. (Adopted unanimously.)
14. No inducements, monetary or otherwise, should be offered to procure an abortion for research purposes. (Adopted unanimously.)
15. Research which is supported by the Secretary, DHEW, to be conducted outside the United States should at the minimum comply in full with the standards and procedures recommended herein. (Adopted unanimously.)

Recommendations Nos. 10 and 11, seek to remove all decisions concerning the abortion from the research protocol, its necessity, method and timing. If a physician is involved in a research program, then decisions as to the health care of the pregnant woman or the fetus must be subjected to the medical judgment of a physician not associated with the program.

The means by which it is assured that health care and research interests do not conflict and that independent medical judgments are offered is the review panel. Hence, provision for such monitoring by the panel should be contained in the prospectus which solicits the grant of funds from DHEW.

In the 12th recommendation, it is stated that research on abortion techniques be continued. In his minority report, Louisell informs us that emotional pleas were "made at the Commission's hearings not to acknowledge limitations on experimentations that would inhibit court-granted permissive abortion."[7] For the most part, he states, the Commission resisted this pressure. "But at the last meeting, without prior preparation or discussion, it adopted recommendation 12, promotive of research on abortion techniques."[8] In Louisell's opinion, this action was imprudent, not germane to the Commission's task, and not adequately considered. Indeed, it is difficult to understand how this recommendation relates to the mandate of the Commission.

The 10th and 12th recommendations were passed by a vote of six to two. Of the 11 individuals on the Commission, three did not vote concerning these important recommendations. Only six individuals—barely a simple majority—approved these recommendations and thus were able to influence the formulation of national policy. In matters of such moment, a greater majority should be required before a proposition is adopted by the Commission. Perhaps in the future a two-thirds majority of the 11-member board should be required to vote affirmatively before a recommendation is approved. Moreover, the number of individuals who abstained from voting, as well as the positive and negative votes, should be identified.

The 13th recommendation states that individuals have a right to refuse to cooperate in the performance of any health service program or research activity contrary to their religious beliefs or moral convictions. It should be specified that the same right should be granted to institutions.

The 14th recommendation prohibits the offering of inducements, monetary or otherwise, to procure abortions for research purposes. Language should be added which would prohibit offering inducements of money for the "products" of abortions, i.e., the abortuses, because of the danger of illicit trafficking in living and dead fetuses. The 15th recommendation requires that research sponsored by DHEW outside the United States also would comply with these standards. These recommendations are worthy ones, but it is not clear as to how they will be enforced. Will the review procedure suffice?

Termination of Moratorium on Fetal Experimentation. In its final recommendation, the Commission asks that the moratorium on fetal experimentation be lifted immediately and that research be allowed to continue under current regulations. It also requests that the recommendations of the Commission be implemented by the DHEW Secretary as soon as public response to them is received and incorporated into the final regulations.

16. The moratorium which is currently in effect should be lifted immediately, allowing research to proceed under current regulations but with the application of the commission's recommendations to the review process. All the foregoing recommendations of the commission should be implemented as soon as the Secretary, DHEW, is able to promulgate regulations based upon these recommendations and the public response to them. (Adopted by a vote of 9 to 1.)

Louisell maintains that requesting an end to the moratorium is "beyond our [the Commission's] control and we ought not assume authority that is not ours. This is matter not for us and not, ultimately, for any administrative official, but for Congress."[9] Louisell's argument is based not only upon the fact that Congress declared the moratorium and therefore should be the agency to lift it, but also upon assertion that the gravity of the action involved, namely, removing "protection of the established principles governing human experimentation," is of such significance that Congress should be the only representative voice that could effect this change in national policy. If one studies the implications of the recommendations, especially those that allow research upon nonconsenting human subjects, the rationale behind Louisell's statement becomes clear. Short of a national referendum, only the Congress as representative of the people, and even then questionably, could make so basic a change in public policy.

This concludes the study of the National Commission's recommendations. Many suggestions have been made in the above text indicating ways of formulating the recommendations which would more fully implement the ethical principles involved. Appendix II of this study contains an alternative formulation of the recommendations which incorporates these suggestions. However, a practical issue remains: that of the actual federal regulations now in effect as a result of the Commission's recommendations.

Review of the Federal Regulations Regarding Fetal Experimentation

Federal regulations governing fetal experimentation became effective on August 8, 1975, some two and one-half months following the submission of the sixteen recommendations (discussed above) by the National Commission for the Protection of Human Subjects of Biomedical and Behavioral Research.

This study will consist of a brief review of these current federal regulations in light of the principles developed in previous sections and chapters. Undoubtedly, these regulations will undergo further modification and refinement as the concerned public makes its views known to the Department of Health, Education and Welfare. But before we examine the actual regulations, however, a brief chronology of their development might be in order.

The first working draft of a policy statement of DHEW regarding additional protection for fetuses, abortuses, pregnant women, and the products of human *in vitro* fertilization was published in November, 1973.[10] Approximately six months later, a policy regarding the protection of *adult* human subjects was published (its provisions to be effective on July 1, 1974), which stated additionally that it was in the process of developing policies to govern research involving the fetus and the abortus.[11] Recognition was given, in addition, to the role and the anticipated recommendations of the newly created National Commission for the Protection of Human Subjects of Biomedical and Behavioral Research.

During its process of framing the recommendations, the National Commission strongly solicited public comment from many and various individuals, organizations and interest groups. This also was the policy of DHEW in its determination of the regulations, and public comment was requested following publication of each draft and policy statement.

Finally, on August 8, 1975, the Department of Health, Education and Welfare published its rules and regulations "governing research involving the fetus, the pregnant woman and the products of human *in vitro* fertilization consistent with the public comments and the Recommendations of the Commission."[13] As was stated previously, these regulations will very likely be modified and refined in accordance with the impact of public opinion as it is made known to the Department.

The Federal Regulations

The revised regulations presented in the *FEDERAL REGISTER* contain a prefatory discussion which should be consulted for a fuller appreciation of the Regulations, as it explains briefly their background within the recommendations of the National Commission and in previous policy.[14]

The regulations will be studied here in eight sections, each followed by a brief selection on significant aspects. Suggested modifications or clarifications of the present Federal Regulations are printed in *italics.*

Ethical Advisory Boards: After stating the definitions previously cited in Chapter I above, the first section describes the establishment of two Ethical Advisory Boards and their specific charge:

§ 46.204 Ethical Advisory Boards.

(a) Two Ethical Advisory Boards shall be established by the Secretary. Members of these Boards shall be so selected that the Boards will be competent to deal with medical, legal, social, ethical, and related issues and may include, for example, research scientists, physicians, psychologists, sociologists, educators, lawyers, and ethicists, as well as representatives of the general public.

No board member may be a regular, full-time employee of the Federal Government.

(b) One Board shall be advisory to the Public Health Service and its components. One Board shall be advisory to all other agencies and components within the Department of Health, Education, and Welfare.

(c) At the request of the Secretary, the appropriate Ethical Advisory Board shall render advice consistent with the policies and requirements of this Part as to ethical issues, involving activities covered by this subpart, raised by individual applications or proposals. In addition, upon request by the Secretary, the appropriate Board shall render advice as to classes of applications or proposals and general policies, guidelines, and procedures.

(d) A Board may establish, with the approval of the Secretary, classes of applications or proposals which: (1) Must be submitted to the Board, or (2) need not be submitted to the Board. Where the Board so establishes a class of applications or proposals which must be submitted, no application or proposal within the class may be funded by the Department or any component thereof until the application or proposal has been reviewed by the Board and the Board has rendered advice as to its acceptability from an ethical standpoint.

(e) No application or proposal involving human *in vitro* fertilization may be funded by the Department or any component thereof until the application or proposal has been reviewed by the Ethical Advisory Board and the Board has rendered advice as to its acceptability from an ethical standpoint.

While the existence of Ethical Advisory Boards may add another burden to research, they may also provide a check on the possible disproportionate influence of a particularly powerful or prominent individual scientist. Further, the Commission recommended adequate representation of women and minorities on such Boards and stipulated that their deliberations be made public. However, there is also the possibility that the power to approve a waiver of specific regulations by the Secretary (of DHEW), as is granted in 46.205, below, could lead to the kind of research the regulations were meant to prohibit. As will be mentioned in a subsequent section, *such waivers should not be permitted since they undermine the ethical norms of the regulations.*

Duties of Institutional Review Boards: The next section (46.205) deals with the additional duties of the local Institutional Review Boards.

§ 46.205 Additional duties of the Institutional Review Boards in connection with activities involving fetuses, pregnant women, or human in vitro fertilization.

(a) In addition to the responsibilities prescribed for Institutional Review Boards under Subpart A of this part, the applicant's or offeror's Board shall, with respect to activities covered by this subpart, carry out the following additional duties:

(1) Determine that all aspects of the activity meet the requirements of this subpart;

(2) Determine that adequate consideration has been given to the manner in which potential subjects will be selected, and adequate provision has been made by the applicant or offeror for monitoring the actual informed consent process (e.g., through such mechanisms, when appropriate, as participation by the Institutional Review Board or subject advocates in: (i) Overseeing the actual process by which individual consents required by this subpart are secured either by approving induction of each individual into the activity or verifying, perhaps through sampling, that approved procedures for induction of individuals into the activity are being followed, and (ii) monitoring the progress of the activity and intervening as necessary through such steps as visits to the activity site and continuing evaluation to determine if any unanticipated risks have arisen);

(3) Carry out such other responsibilities as may be assigned by the Secretary.

(b) No award may be issued until the applicant or offeror has certified to the Secretary that the Institutional Review Board has made the determinations required under paragraph (a) of this section and the Secretary has approved these determinations, as provided in § 46.115 of Subpart A of this part.

(c) Applicants or offerors seeking support for activities covered by this subpart must provide for the designation of an Institutional Review Board, subject to approval by the Secretary, where no such Board has been established under Subpart A of this part.

Institutional Review Boards have already been operative in many medical schools and hospitals. An overall appraisal of such Boards would have to admit a great variation in the manner in which they function and a varying degree of success in the discharge of their responsibilities. Although the effectiveness of these federal regulations in protecting the basic rights of the humans who are research subjects ultimately rests on the ethical probity of those conducting the research, the existence of these Institutional Review Boards does act as a reminder and confronter. Experience, however, supports the view that the effectiveness of these Boards depends in large measure on the commitment of its chairperson and on the degree of support he or she, and the work of the Board, receive from the highest administrative or executive officer of their particular institution.

One of the major ambiguities in the federal regulations surrounds the concept of "minimal risk." Not only are there no criteria proposed for ascertaining the range of risks that might be considered "minimal," but there is reason for concern that, no matter what standards are devised, their application to fetuses designated for abortion, or who were electively aborted, might well differ from the application to those fetuses who will be carried to term. It would seem appropriate, then, that the regulations include a mandate to the local Institutional Review Committee *requiring that it specify and stringently require uniform application of adequate safeguards in the determination of minimal risk.*

General Limitations: Having dealt with Advisory and Review Boards, the next section now considers several limiting conditions to fetal research:

> **§ 46.206 General limitations.**
>
> (a) No activity to which this subpart is applicable may be undertaken unless:
>
> (1) Appropriate studies on animals and nonpregnant individuals have been completed;
>
> (2) Except where the purpose of the activity is to meet the health needs of the particular fetus, the risk to the fetus is minimal and, in all cases, is the least possible risk for achieving the objectives of the activity;
>
> (3) Individuals engaged in the activity will have no part in: (i) Any decisions as to the timing, method, and procedures used to terminate the pregnancy, and (ii) determining the viability of the fetus at the termination of the pregnancy; and
>
> (4) No procedural changes which may cause greater than minimal risk to the fetus or the pregnant woman will be introduced into the procedure for terminating the pregnancy solely in the interest of the activity.
>
> (b) No inducements, monetary or otherwise, may be offered to terminate pregnancy for purposes of the activity.

The listed limitations are all genuinely concerned with protecting the dignity of the fetus even though current laws permit widespread abortion. An attempt is made to keep distinct these two issues by insisting that those engaged in fetal experimentation not be involved in the decision to abort (Nos. 3,4). Yet, these rules obviously presuppose the ready availability of abortuses. Despite the good intention of these limitations, they may actually encourage abortions by enveloping that procedure with an aura of respectability and worth in the form of medical benefits to the class of fetuses. In addition, there is the danger, already mentioned above, that the evaluation of minimal risk will be differentially applied to fetuses about to be aborted and to fetuses destined for survival by human choice. *To protect the equality of fetuses with one another, risk should be judged on the basis of the generalized class of fetuses of comparable age and development.* The fact that abortion is anticipated or already begun should not modify the risk estimate for any given fetus. The principle of equality cannot otherwise be preserved in practice.

Pregnant women as research subjects: Following these general considerations, the subsequent section of the Regulations considers those research activities directed toward pregnant women:

> **§ 46.207 Activities directed toward pregnant women as subjects.**
>
> (a) No pregnant woman may be involved as a subject in an activity covered by this subpart unless: (1) The purpose of the activity is to meet the health needs of the mother and the fetus will be placed at risk only to the minimum extent necessary to meet such needs, or (2) the risk to the fetus is minimal.
>
> (b) An activity permitted under paragraph (a) of this section may be conducted only if the mother and father are legally competent and have given their informed consent after having been fully informed regarding possible impact on the fetus, except that the father's informed consent need not be secured if: (1) The purpose of the activity is to meet the health needs of the mother; (2) his identity or whereabouts cannot reasonably be ascertained; (3) he is not reasonably available; or (4) the pregnancy resulted from rape.

Part (a) of this regulation is concerned with the pregnant woman as the subject of a research medical procedure directed to benefit her life and health. A problem arises in the balancing of the woman's health needs with the degree of risk to which the fetus would be concurrently exposed. *No statement is made as to a proportionality that should exist between the health needs of the mother and the wellbeing of the unborn infant.* Further, if the fetus is destined for abortion, there is a danger that he/she would be exposed to greater additional injury than would otherwise have been considered acceptable.

The second part (b) of that section introduces a departure from the Commission's recommendations. The latter had only stated that "the father had not objected." However, DHEW rightly insists that *paternal* consent *be requested,* allowing, however, for some specific exceptions. This is a reasonable provision inasmuch as the father has an obligation to protect the life and health of his children.

Fetuses in utero as research subjects: In this section, the focus of the research is not the pregnant woman but the fetus still *in utero:*

> **§ 46.208 Activities directed toward fetuses in utero as subjects.**
>
> (a) No fetus *in utero* may be involved as a subject in any activity covered by this subpart unless: (1) The purpose of the

activity is to meet the health needs of the particular fetus and the fetus will be placed at risk only to the minimum extent necessary to meet such needs, or (2) the risk to the fetus imposed by the research is minimal and the purpose of the activity is the development of important biomedical knowledge which cannot be obtained by other means.

(b) An activity permitted under paragraph (a) of this section may be conducted only if the mother and father are legally competent and have given their informed consent, except that the father's consent need not be secured if: (1) His identity or whereabouts cannot reasonably be ascertained, (2) he is not reasonably available, or (3) the pregnancy resulted from rape.

Since in this section no distinction is made as to whether the fetus in question is destined to go to term or to be aborted, the presumption should be clarified that no such distinction will be countenanced here. *It should be noted that no provision is made in (a) (1) for the wellbeing of the mother, yet the risk to her should not exceed the expected benefit for the fetus.*

The provision in (a) (2) contains a second ambiguity, comparable to that surrounding "minimal risk," with the phrase "development of important biomedical knowledge which cannot be obtained by other means." First, what criteria are to be used in ascertaining what is "important biomedical knowledge," and second, how is it to be established that other means are not available? Admittedly, it is difficult, even retrospectively, to determine that a particular medical discovery could have been reached by other means than those actually employed. However, in the face of an urgent problem needing solution, the temptation should be resisted of employing a live human fetus for a research activity (if little effort or thought was expended in searching for alternate means) without first exhausting alternative means of obtaining the desired information.

Premature surviving and nonsurviving infants as research subjects: The regulations in this section review the conditions necessary for involving premature infants in research:

§ 46.209 Activities directed toward fetuses ex utero, including nonviable fetuses, as subjects.

(a) No fetus *ex utero* may be involved as a subject in an activity covered by this subpart until it has been ascertained whether the particular fetus is viable, unless: (1) There will be no added risk to the fetus resulting from the activity, and (2) the purpose of the activity is the development of important biomedical knowledge which cannot be obtained by other means.

(b) No nonviable fetus may be involved as a subject in an activity covered by this subpart unless: (1) Vital functions of the fetus will not be artificially maintained except where the purpose of the activity is to develop new methods for enabling fetuses to survive to the point of viability, (2) experimental activities which of themselves would terminate the heartbeat or respiration of the fetus will not be employed, and (3) the purpose of the activity is the development of important biomedical knowledge which cannot be obtained by other means.

(c) In the event the fetus *ex utero* is found to be viable, it may be included as a subject in the activity only to the extent permitted by and in accordance with the requirements of other subparts of this part.

(d) An activity permitted under paragraph (a) or (b) of this section may be conducted only if the mother and father are legally competent and have given their informed consent, except that the father's informed consent need not be secured if: (1) his identity or whereabouts cannot reasonably be ascertained, (2) he is not reasonably available, or (3) the pregnancy resulted from rape.

The first provision of this regulation requires that it first be determined whether or not the fetus *ex utero* is viable. According to the DHEW's definition, the fetus is deemed viable if it is able "to survive (given the benefit of available medical therapy) to the point of independently maintaining heartbeat and respiration."[16] Hence, the provision clearly provides that an effort be made to keep the fetus alive, because, without such effort, it could not honestly be said that the fetus was either viable or nonviable. *This provision should be strengthened with the insistence that every reasonable effort be made to maintain life in the fetus.*

The two provisions in the latter part of (a) seem to allow neglect in attempting to maintain the life of the fetus *if* there is no added risk to the fetus from the experimental procedure and important knowledge is at stake. The two provisions seem quite reasonable, but only in conjunction with responsible efforts to preserve the life of the fetus *ex utero.* Half-hearted attempts to utilize appropriate life sustaining measures may be related to the commonly held notion that notably premature infants are not worth saving because they will most likely be afflicted with some significant abnormality. However, recent studies seem to demonstrate the critical factor to be perinatal care, and that, with quality medical and nursing care, these infants, with regard to frequency of abnormalities, are no different than their full-term counterparts.[17]

Serious objections have been raised to the provision in (b)(1) which permits the continued artificial maintenance of vital functions in a definitely *nonviable* fetus for the purpose of developing new methods of bringing other fetuses to the point of viability. As noble as the goal may be, the utilization of *nonviable* fetuses for such a purpose is clearly to use a human subject without appropriate informed consent for the benefit of another. In such a situation a person is used as a *pure means* for the welfare of others. This is contrary to the inherent dignity of a human subject as developed in Chapters II, III and IV. Indeed, the National Commission so strenuously objected to this provision that Dr. Cooper, the

Assistant Secretary for Health, stated that new regulations would be drafted limiting research studies on nonviable fetuses *ex utero* to those in which there was some hope of benefit to the particular fetus.[18]

In this connection, it seems preferable to designate possibly-viable fetuses as the more appropriate subjects for experiments directed to aid premature infants to survive. Granted, it may be a difficult medical decision in particular cases to determine whether a premature infant has at least a remote chance of survival, even with the aid of heroic life sustaining procedures. Nonetheless, it seems incumbent on the physician-investigator to test out new procedures and equipment directed to bring a premature infant to the point where he or she can independently maintain pulmonary and cardiovascular functions, only on those premature infants who have some possiblity of survival. In such cases, the research would really be of a therapeutic nature since the hope and intention was to help this particular fetus as well as others in his/her class.

Use of fetal material and dead fetuses: In this section, provision is made to employ fetus-related tissues for research studies:

§ 46.210 Activities involving the dead fetus, fetal material, or the placenta.

Activities involving the dead fetus, mascerated fetal material, or cells, tissue, or organs excised from a dead fetus shall be conducted only in accordance with any applicable State or local laws regarding such activities.

It can be granted that the dead fetus is no longer a human subject in the proper sense, and it can be granted even further that a dead fetus is no fetus at all but rather an agglomeration of tissues and cells which convey only the *appearance* of a fetus since they lack the functional integrity of a (living) fetus. Nonetheless, the corporeal remains of fetuses merit true respect because of their previous association with a human spirit.

Waiver of Specific Requirements: This final section of the Regulations provides the process by which an institution can seek to have a particular requirement waived.

§ 46.211 Modification or waiver of specific requirements.

Upon the request of an applicant or offeror (with the approval of its Institutional Review Board), the Secretary may modify or waive specific requirements of this subpart, with the approval of the Ethical Advisory Board after such opportunity for public comment as the Ethical Advisory Board considers appropriate in the particular instance. In making such decisions, the Secretary will consider whether the risks to the subject are so outweighed by the sum of the benefit to the subject and the importance of the knowledge to be gained as to warrant such modification or waiver and that such benefits cannot be gained except through a modification or waiver. Any such modifications or waivers will be published as notices in the FEDERAL REGISTER.

This provision could well open a regulatory "Pandora's Box." Even with the checks and restraining influence of the local Institutional Review Board and of the National Ethical Review Board, the possibility for arbitrary judgment and thus for abuse remains open. As the Secretary has the power, with concurrence of the Boards, to render inoperative one or more of these regulations in particular instances, possible pressure created by persons strongly professing some alleged biomedical advancement might well make it possible for a fetus to be deprived of all protection. Expediency could override ethical concerns and the requirements of proxy consent. It is stipulated that waivers or modifications would be published as notices in the *Federal Register.* But it is questionable whether notice by such *post factum* publications would constitute an effective restraining measure. Therefore, the permission of such waivers should not be considered and the ambiguous statement allowing the Secretary to consider the sum of benefit to the subject and the importance of such knowledge to be gained should be dropped. The Ethical Advisory Board should be consulted, though, in areas where it should review local decisions to permit experimentation in the face of advocacy of the rights of the fetus. (See Item (3)(b) in the "Essential Elements for Alternative Regulations" below.)

Proposed Essential Elements for Alternative Regulations

Any federal regulation should properly consider the legitimate interests and rights of those who will experience the effects of the regulations most directly. At the same time, the nature and concerns of the society at large which provides financial support for the activities to be regulated must also be borne in mind. It is with these concerns in mind, and against the background of the discussions in the preceding chapters, that the following, rather concise set of elements for alternative regulations has been prepared. Even though they may never be fully incorporated into federal regulations, these alternative regulations would seem to be dictated by the considerations presented above in Chapters I through VI. Thus, they would seem appropriate for Catholic hospitals and researchers as well as for all other institutions and individuals who concur with the analysis above.

The primary actors in the arena of fetal experimentation are: (1) the fetus, (2) the mother (and the father), (3) the researcher, including the supporting staff and the institution in which the research is being carried out. More remotely involved are the class of infants who will ultimately benefit from the research findings, and still more remote to the action are various segments of the public who in some way are indirectly related to the activity and may finance it by tax money.

As was previously emphasized, the principal concern of any regulation should be to protect the rights and to promote the legitimate interests of those involved. Accordingly, the following elements should be included in any regulations designed to govern fetal research.

1. Concerning the fetus:
   a. He/she has a basic right to life and health; hence, both prior to and following delivery, no research activity may be undertaken which jeopardizes the health or life of the fetus.
   b. In assessing the risk of harm, no distinction should be made between the aborted fetus, or the one designated for abortion, or the one being brought to term.
   c. If a pregnant woman is the subject of a procedure directed to her health needs, due proportion should be observed between the degree of risk to which the fetus will be exposed and the expected benefit to the mother.
   d. If a pregnant woman is the subject of a research procedure which is not directed to her health needs, the risk to the fetus must be minimal.
   e. No living fetus *in utero* nor any living fetus *ex utero,* that is, a premature infant, will be the subject of a research activity unless it is directed to his/her benefit, or entails no, or minimal, risk.[19] Research protocols should give evidence of their assessment of risk involved and the criteria employed. Evidence of obvious discomfort of a fetus, whether *in utero* or *ex utero,* or of any significant interference with bodily or functional integrity should be considered a *prima facie* indication of more than minimal risk. Institutional Review Boards should consider carefully the criteria and estimate of risk in protocols reviewed.
   f. The fetus *ex utero,* that is, a premature infant, should not be judged as incapable of sustaining vital functions until this has been established by the failure of suitably employed artificial life support systems.
2. Concerning the mother (and father):
   a. In all instances of research activity involving a fetus, informed consent will be obtained from the mother except when she has granted permission for an elective abortion. In the latter case, informed consent must be obtained from a court-appointed guardian.
   b. Similarly, informed consent must be obtained from the father except in those cases where the health needs of the mother are involved or he cannot be contacted after a reasonable effort.

3. Concerning the researcher:
   a. The persons conducting a research activity directed to the fetus shall not participate in decisions regarding the time, method, or procedures to be used in an abortion, nor will such be involved in the determination of a fetus' capability to be maintained on artificial life support systems to the point of independently sustaining vital functions.
   b. When a conflict arises between what a researcher deems as an appropriate research procedure directed toward a fetus and the well-being of the fetus, as represented in writing by any interested advocate of the fetus, the Institutional Review Board—which should have appropriate representation from the concerned community—will resolve the issue and forward their decision to the National Ethical Advisory Board for review.

Summary

Current federal policy emanates from the Report and Recommendations of the National Commission for the Protection of Human Subjects of Biomedical and Behavioral Research and is reflected in the regulations published by the Department of Health, Education and Welfare based on the Commission's Report. A careful critique of the Commission's Report showed much that is ethically acceptable and laudable but in at least one recommendation (No. 6) a fetus of less than 20 weeks gestational age is left with minimal protection. Numerous other points of possible ambiguous interpretation are also noted.

The federal regulations which were published on August 8, 1975 were based on an earlier policy that had been modified by comments from the public and by the Commission's Recommendations. A careful review of these regulations revealed some departures from the Commission's Report as well as some provisions that were deemed incompatible with the principles developed in this study. In one instance, however, while the Department of Health, Education and Welfare's initial regulations appear to permit keeping a fetus alive for the sole purpose of research, recent objections, including some from members of the Commission, will apparently result in the banning of nontherapeutic research on the nonviable fetus (i.e., the living, premature infant not capable of prolonged extrauterine life). The possible ambiguities of the present regulations led the authors of this study to offer constructive suggestions in their reflections on the various sections of the Regulations. This chapter concludes with some suggested elements which are directed to eliminate these defects in a simplified and coherent way and to provide the basis for a more acceptable set of guidelines.

Conclusion

This lengthy chapter on the work of the National Commission for the Protection of Human Subjects of Biomedical and Behavioral Research and on the current regulations of the Department of Health, Education and Welfare should not be construed as opposing the main thrust of these efforts, which are clearly commendable and ethically valuable. Nonetheless, to some persons in the general public, the regulations may appear to be too severe.

The authors of this study are convinced that the substance of the current Federal Regulations conforms to the conclusions pertaining to the core ethical issues in fetal experimentation as developed in Chapter V from the previous consensus on the intrinsic human dignity of the fetus as outlined in Chapters II, III and IV. In particular, the substance of the seven summary propositions in Chapter V at the conclusion of the section of "Fetal Experimentation and Community Ethical Values" can be found in the present Federal Regulations. These Regulations *do* seek to respect the ethical norm that proxy consent cannot be given for nontherapeutic fetal experimentation which involves more than minimal risk to the fetus. And they *do,* implicitly at least, prohibit discrimination between the treatment of fetuses who will be aborted or have been aborted and other fetuses who will be brought to term.

However, as the comments in the reflections above on each section of the Federal Regulations indicate, further clarifications should be made in the Federal Regulations. Copies of this study have been sent to the Department of Health, Education and Welfare. Readers of this study who concur with the clarifications suggested here, or who may wish to express their convictions with regard to other aspects of human experimentation, may do so by sending their comments and appropriate documentation to the following address:

Office of Protection from Research Risks
National Institutes of Health
9000 Rockville Pike
Bethesda, Maryland 20014

Finally, as mentioned above, the proposed elements for alternative regulations suggested here do have the advantage of presenting in a concise and comparatively simple fashion the full ethical norms proposed above in Chapter V. The Pope John XXIII Center offers these alternative and simplified elements in the sincere hope that they will assist individual researchers and research institutions in pursuing fetal research according to the humanism of the Judaeo-Christian heritage and its parallel in those expressions of secular humanism which recognize the intrinsic dignity of all human subjects.

CHAPTER VI Footnotes

1. For a brief explanation of how this commission came into being, consult Ramsey, Paul, *The Ethics of Fetal Research,* New Haven, Connecticut: Yale University Press, 1975.

2. "Protection of Human Subjects:, *Federal Register* 40(154): 33530–33551, August 8, 1975.
3. Louisell, David, "Fetal Research: A Dissent", *Origins,* June 12, 1975, p. 43.
4. *Ibid.*
5. Ibid., p. 44.
6. In his testimony, speaking on behalf of the United States Catholic Conference, Msgr. James McHugh urged "a general disposition against experiments on dead fetuses after abortion because in light of the value judgment reached by the U. S. Supreme Court in *Wade and Bolton,* the human fetus *can too easily be reduced* to the status of an experimental animal." (The National Commission for the Protection of Human Subjects of Biomedical and Behavioral Research, Verbatim Report, February 14-15, 1975, p. 211.)
7. *Op. cit,* p. 44.
8. *Ibid.*
9. *Op. cit., . 45.*
10. Federal Register 38(221):31738, November 16, 1973.
11. *Federal Register* 39(105):18914, May 30, 1974.
12. *Federal Register* 39(165):30648, August 23, 1974.
13. *Federal Register* 40(154):33526, August 8, 1975.
14. *Ibid.,* p. 33526-33528
15. *Ibid.,* p. 33527.
16. *Ibid.,* p. 33529.
17. See George Cassady, "Impact of Neonatal Intensive Care on Quality of Life", *Clinical Perinatology,* edited by S. Hadjen and Audrey K. Brown, St. Louis: C. V. Mosby, Inc., 1974, pp. 422–438.
18. "The Blue Sheet", *Drug Research Reports,* 18(51), December 17, 1975.
19. It must be emphatically stated that whatever procedure is envisaged, in no way should it be harmful to the fetus. This point is well developed by Hans O. Tiefel, "The Cost of Fetal Research: Ethical Considerations," *New England Journal of Medicine* 294(2):85–90, January 8, 1976.

Epilogue

The ethical implications of fetal experimentation have been analyzed in the context of the civic community, of personalist humanism, and of Christian belief. The key issues of consent and minimal risk have been explored and a careful analysis has manifested some ambivalence in the Recommendations of the National Commission and in the Federal Regulations. Suggested modifications based on the analysis in this study have been proposed.

This study concludes now with two additional major objectives still to be attained, the first of these being that of persuading the scientific research community to accept the limitations proposed above on non-therapeutic fetal research. Obviously, the scientific advances which could be made with the unlimited use of fetal subjects are potentially great, as they would be with the unlimited use of adult subjects. The objection, however, would be the same in both cases: scientific progress would have been made at the cost of undermining human values and of involving the exploitation of human persons.

As indicated in the introduction to this study, the *need* for non-therapeutic research *is not absolute, but relative.* Significant progress has been, and will continue to be made in the overcoming of birth deformities and in developing a scientific fetology without resorting to the exploitation of living fetuses. Scientific research will more likely benefit because of increased social support which might otherwise diminish if the public felt that science were no longer a servant.

Effectively persuading the research community to preserve the intrinsic dignity of fetal subjects will depend heavily on the second unfinished task - the establishment of a consensus in the American community that recognizes the intrinsic dignity of the entire class of human fetuses. The converging argumentation presented in this study is not presently a matter of full consensus or even of adequate dialogue among responsible community leaders. Because of the emotionally explosive abortion debate, many sincere persons harbor many doubts as to the proper degree of human dignity and the nature of human rights to be accorded human fetuses. However, we are confident that if the reasoning offered in this study is fully aired in public dialogue, a stronger consensus will emerge.

The Pope John XXIII Medical-Moral Research and Education Center has prepared this study to explore the issue of fetal research both in the light of Catholic doctrine and of generally accepted humanistic values. These suggested revisions of the Federal Regulations are dictated both by Catholic teaching and responsible contemporary humanism. We offer this study in the hope of furthering the process of Christian/humanist dialogue that is so essential to the development of appropriate public policy in our pluralistic society.

It is our hope that the considerations here presented will influence scientific investigators as they design research protocols in pursuit of their important goals of expanding medical knowledge and improving therapeutic procedures. Furthermore, we trust that it will contribute to the enhancement of society's commitment to the continued well-being of the human community, which depends ultimately on its respect for the rights of all its members.

Appendix I

A Critique of the Theory of Delayed Hominization

by Benedict Ashley, O.P.

St. Thomas Aquinas, following Aristotle, argued that the human embryo is at first alive only with vegetative life, then with animal or sensitive life, and only after at least 40 days of development is it prepared to become a human person by receiving a human, intellective soul from the Creator. Consequently, induced abortion before 40 days is a serious "sin against nature," because it destroys an organism whose natural purpose is to be transformed into a human being, but such abortion is not, strictly speaking, homicide.[1]

Strangely, this medieval theory is again the subject of discussion among Catholic theologians, in spite of the fact that they are eager, since Vatican II, to free their thinking from a rigid, "official" Thomism. Although ultimately the authoritative position of the Catholic Church does not rest on the acceptance or rejection of this particular theory (Chapter IV, pp. 81–87), it requires careful examination, even at the cost of some scholastic subtleties, for two reasons.

First, because in the casuistic technique of traditional Catholic moral theology, weight is always given to traditional positions of notable authorities, even when these opinions appear to have only an extrinsic value, somewhat as in arguing from legal precedents. According to the principle of casuistic *probablism,* it is safe in practice to follow such solidly probable opinions, even when the opposite view is more probable.

Consequently, a number of responsible moral theologians in recent publications have adduced the authority of Aquinas, of Alphonsus Ligouri, and numerous other "standard authors" to argue that there is solid probability that induced abortion in the earliest period of pregnancy is not homicide, and consequently in a conflict of rights that involves grave risk to the life of the mother (or an equivalent risk), the rights of the mother, who is certainly human, may be preferred against those of the child who is probably not human in the earliest period of pregnancy.[2]

Second, Fr. Joseph Donceel, S.J., in several influential articles, has not only strengthened this argument from authority by showing that the opposite view arose in the church in the seventeenth century, largely through the influence of Cartesian dualism, but has gone on to argue the validity of Aquinas' theory of "mediate animation" (or "delayed hominization", as Donceel more accurately names it) on its own intrinsic merits.[3] He believes that when Aquinas' theory has been freed from medieval biology it remains valid as a philosophical theory, and when this theory is used to interpret the data of modern embryology, we can conclude with high probability, even certainty, that the embryo in its first three months of existence cannot be a human person. The only solid reason, therefore, for opposing abortion during this period is that this is a "sin against nature." Donceel is not alone in his views, which have been supported by Fr. Plé, O.P., and by two Catholic physicians, James J. Diamond, M.D. and Bernard J. Ransil, M.D.[4]

On the contrary, I will argue that if the philosophical principles of Aquinas are correctly applied to the data of modern embryology, the theory of delayed hominization turns out to be quite implausible. Consequently, we must judge the traditional authority for this view in Catholic moral theology to be obsolete, since it would appear from the history of the question as outlined by Donceel himself, that St. Thomas' defense of the theory was not only the most influential, but also the strongest on its merits.

Fr. Donceel's argument is stated by him succinctly as follows:

> Philosophically speaking, we can be certain that an organism is a human person only from its activities. The most typically human activity is reflection, self-awareness, the power of saying, "I." Of course, if we had to wait until a child starts to say "I" or to use the word "true" (which implies some self-reflection), we would have to delay hominization until longer after birth. The Church has condemned this position (DS 2135) and rightly so. When we sleep or have fainted, we possess no self-awareness either, yet we remain human beings; we remain capable of such activities. A person in the ultimate stage of senility may give no more sign of self-awareness, yet he still possesses the organs required for such activity. The least we may ask before admitting the presence of a human soul is the availability of these organs: the senses, the nervous system, the brain and especially the cortex. Since these organs are not ready during early pregnancy,

I feel certain that there is no human person until several weeks have elapsed.[5]

He bases this argument on the Thomistic principle that since the human soul, although spiritual, is created by God as the substantial form of the human body, it can only inform matter sufficiently prepared for ensoulment, and this requires that this matter have: (a) a differentiation into organs, including (b) the proper organ of man's highest animal activities (the "internal senses"), which, according to modern understanding, must be the cerebral cortex.[6] He gives little attention to St. Thomas' concern with the question of the *efficient cause* of the preparation of the matter, although historically this is the principal question for Aquinas.[7] For Donceel the issue is simply that of the relation of the material to the efficient cause. We can formulate his essential argument thus:

Hominization is possible only when there exists the organ (i.e., the actual capability) required for the specifically human operations of thought and will.

This organ is the brain, and probably the cerebral cortex.

Therefore, hominization is possible only when there exists the brain, or better, the cerebral cortex.

I would concede the major premise of this argument, at least as a correct statement of Aquinas' hylomorphic philosophy of the unity of the human person, but I would distinguish the minor by substituting for "cerebral cortex" the expression "the epigenetic primordium (anlage) of the cerebral cortex." Clearly Donceel himself does not mean that the cerebral cortex in its full mature development must be present, since this would bring hominization to a post-natal period, but only that it must be present in some way that we can empirically verify its radical identity with the mature cortex. As he grants, it need not be actually operational.

Our problem, therefore, becomes to determine on the basis of current data at what point in embryonic development this radical identity can be verified. Since preformationist theories of embryology are not scientifically acceptable today, and are certainly inconsistent with hylomorphism, what we are trying to determine is the epigenetic, and not the preformed, origin of the cortex.

Following Aquinas' line of thought, then, what results do we arrive at in view of current data? The response to that query will be divided into three major sections: a) The meaning and implications of this Thomistic theory; b) An evaluation of this theory in light of current embryological data; and c) A brief consideration of three objections commonly brought forward against immediate hominization.

The Meaning and Implications of this Thomistic Theory

1) *What degree of preparation of the matter did Aquinas require for its union with the spiritual soul to be hylomorphically possible?* To answer

this, we must understand the epigenetic theory of embryology, which Aquinas derived from Aristotle.[8]

The basic axiom of Aristotle's philosophy of nature is that "whatever is moved is moved by another." At first sight the living organism seems to defy this law, because a living thing is precisely a substance which is self-moving, self-developing, self-reproductive. This self-activity is the empirical evidence that a thing is alive and ensouled, since by "soul" we simply mean the form of a material thing that is self-active. The different species of living things are specified and recognized precisely by different kinds of such self-activity. Man is man and is recognized to be such by the fact that he has characteristic human self-activities, such as speech, invention, free choice.

The soul of a living thing, however, is its principle as a formal cause, not as an efficient cause. It is only by mediation of its parts, each informed by a vital "power" (which is to the part, as the soul is to the whole organism) that a living thing moves itself, one part moving another. Consequently, in every living being there must be parts, and these (unlike the parts of inanimate chemical substances) must be heterogeneous, at least to the extent that one part is active and the other passive, so that the organism can move itself with the active part used to move the passive part. This active part is the *primary* part; and the passive part is, at first, in the embryological development of the organism, undifferentiated. The organism develops *epigenetically* because of this original lack of differentiation. (In the theory of *preformism* the parts would exist in differentiation from the start, but in miniature.)

However, from the beginning this primary part must exist not only as actually differentiated but must also be actively efficient (i.e., it must be not only in "first act" but also in "second act") because it is the "prime mover" of the whole organic system, without which it could not be alive, nor develop to maturity. The organism is ensouled and alive at the instant when this primary part first appears and begins to act, and it dies when the primary part ceases to act and is destroyed.

Aristotle, however, did not mean by this that when the primary organ first appears, it is itself fully developed in its own structure, nor that it already has its highest and specifically characteristic functions. He had done embryological experiments with fertilized chicken-eggs, and he knew (that the heart which he regarded as the primary organ of animal life that in maturity would be the energetic source of the specifying activity of the animal) first appeared in the chicken egg simply as a pulsating red spot. As this primary organ is the agent which causes the formation of all the other parts of the organism, it also constructs itself. We must assume that it first appears in rudimentary form as a "primordium" which causes the differentiation of its other parts. Thus the primary organ is first present in very simple form and as it constructs the total organism, it also constructs itself in mature form. Similarly, at maturity, this primary organ will be the source of the total activity of the organism, including its highest specifying functions. Thus Aristotle knew that some animals are born before they are able to exercise all characteristic functions proper to their species, especially of sensing and moving; and in all animals the power of reproduction is possible only when the animal approaches maturity.

Thus we can answer our initial question by saying that the human matter is sufficiently prepared for the human soul, when and only when the primary organ of the human body is actually present and beginning to perform its vital functions, but that (a) the other parts need not be differentiated; (b) the primary organ need be present only in primordial form; (c) it need only be functioning to bring about the embryological development of itself and the whole, while its ultimate highest and specifying functions may still be in abeyance, awaiting the various auxiliary organs necessary for such functioning. Finally, we must note that the primary organ, even when it is acting at this more primitive level of functioning, is still acting specifically in a manner characteristic of the species of the organism, since, according to the Aristotelian dictum, "an activity is specified by its term"; hence, since the primary organ is at work building a chicken, a dog, or a human being, its functioning is already the activity of a chicken, dog or human.

2) *Why, then, did Aristotle and Aquinas doubt that the primary organ of human life, and hence the human soul, was present even in primordial form earlier than 40 days of pregnancy?*

Aquinas' doubts, at least, were not based on any idea that the primary organ of human life had to be very large or evidently elaborated. This is clear from the fact that he believed that in the case of the conception of Jesus by the Holy Spirit, hominization took place simultaneously with conception.[9] This was possible because the infinite power of the Holy Spirit was able to complete this necessary preparation of the matter in an instant. However, Aquinas concedes that, at this point, the quantity of Christ's body was very small, and it would be grotesque to suppose that Aquinas imagined this in some preformist, rather than in an epigenetic manner.[10]

Rather, the problem raised for Aquinas was that in non-miraculous conceptions, the efficient cause which must prepare the matter is a finite agent, i.e., the male parent.[11] Such a finite agent can bring about the formation of matter only through a sequence of changes which require some appreciable time. Now, according to the data available to Aristotle, the matter in question was the menstrual blood of the mother. The less organized this matter, the longer time would be required for the agent to carry out the series of steps necessary to prepare it for the human soul.

Aquinas explicitly discusses this question, and concludes that the menstrual blood is an inanimate chemical mixture of nutritional materials in the mother's body which has not been assimilated as an actual part of her living substance, but which has undergone digestive modifications until it is proximately prepared for such assimilation. Thus the efficient cause has the task of raising non-living material to the very high state of organization required to be suitable for the human body. In Aquinas' opinion the flesh of the human body has to have the highest possible type of chemical balance or "temperament," the reason for this being that a sense organ can operate only if it is so tempered that it is neutral to all the contrary qualities found in sensible objects, since if it were colored red, it could not be sensitive to green, or if it were hot, it could not be sensitive to cold, or if hard, to softness. This must be particularly true of the "internal senses" of imagination, etc. which are the necessary instruments of human thinking and willing, since these must be so delicately neutral as to be able to receive a limitless variety of images.[12]

Thus Aristotle and Aquinas could only conclude that the formative action of the male parent would have to take place over a considerable period of time before it could temper the menstrual blood to the level of organization required for a human body that would be capable of the highest type of sensitive life.

3) *How was the manner in which the male parent carries on this formative action conceived?*

The answer to this question is crucial to the plausibility of the delayed hominization theory, yet its defenders have largely neglected it. For Aristotle and Aquinas, it is the major question. In fact this whole embryological question concerns Aquinas mainly because he wishes to refute the *traducianist* theory which holds that the father transmits original sin to his children because the father begets the souls of his children, infecting them with his own sinfulness. Aquinas insists that because the human soul is spiritual it cannot be produced or infused by any material, biological process, but must be immediately created by God (a view which has become authoritative for the Catholic Church).[13] At the same time he is concerned to maintain that both male and female parents are true generators of their offspring, otherwise the doctrine of original sin would lose all meaning, and also the Incarnate Christ would not be truly a member of the human race.[14]

Consequently, Aquinas denies that the human father produces the human soul. Therefore, neither does the father bring about the *ultimate* formation of the matter of the human body, since this is effected by God alone in the very act of creating the soul as the substantial form of the body. What the father does is to bring the menstrual matter to the stage of organization just prior to its hominization, i.e., to a higher level of sensitive life. Because the father himself is infected by original sin his generative activity is in some measure defective, so that this work falls somewhat short of producing a completely "normal" body. Therefore, the soul created for such a body itself suffers infection with original sin from the body. Thus the transmission of human life in the defective condition we call "original sin" is due to the defective action of the male parent.[15]

The male parent, however, is not able directly to act on the menstrual matter because he is not in bodily contact with it, since it exists as unassimilated nutritional material within the mother's body. According to Aristotelian philosophy, no material efficient cause can act on another body except when the two bodies are in actual contact ("no action at a distance"), unless it acts through a "separated" instrument (i.e., another material body which acts as a medium of its efficient action). Aquinas, following Aristotle, believed this instrument of the male agent was the semen. Like the menstrual blood, the semen was not itself alive, but only highly digested nutritional material ready to be assimilated but set aside in the body for another use. It consisted of two portions. One was merely an inactive fluid which, after intercourse, became mixed with the menstrual blood and constituted the male contribution (a minimal one compared with that of the mother's).[16] The other, active portion was a "vital spirit" which was the actual instrument of the male efficiency.[17]

The term "spirit" here does not mean that the active semen was a spiritual entity. Aristotelian biology (also reinforced after Aristotle's time by Stoic theories) thought that living bodies contain various "spirits" which were like hot, energetic gases (or even like our idea of electricity). This seminal spirit, of its own nature, had a high degree of the quality of "heat" and its proper efficient action was to act on the menstrual blood and refine it, just as it was thought that the heat of the body could digest nutritional material. As such, its action was purely chemical, and not strictly vital. However, as an instrument of the male parent, this spirit had been modified in the parent's body so as to have a much more specific efficiency by which it was capable of forming the menstrual blood to the specific neutral temperament required for the human body. This modification of the active semen constituted it a vital instrument, endowed with an intrinsic vital power (*virtus*).[18]

Once the semen had been discharged in the maternal vagina, the passive portion was absorbed, but the active spirit remained as an independent agent acting on the menstrual blood. For Aquinas' theory this was necessary, since "a thing cannot move itself," therefore the agent forming the menstrual blood had to remain separated from, but yet in contact with it. Consequently Aquinas believed that the *semen remained as an active substance throughout the whole period* of preformation of the menstrual matter up to the point of hominization by the creative action of God. The proponents of delayed hominization have failed to notice that this is indispensable to the consistency of his theory.[19]

Is there any alternative which would be consistent with his philosophical principles? It would seem that one might be proposed. It is well known that in applying the notion of instrumental causality to the case of the falling body, and also the projectile, later scholasticism invented the *impetus* theory.[20] Aristotle and Aquinas, in order to preserve the principles "No action at a distance" and "Nothing is moved without a mover distinct from itself," argued that although a projectile is set in motion by the projector, it can continue in motion only because it continues to be moved by the surrounding medium which, unlike the projectile, still has contact with the projector and acts under its influence as its instrument. From the time of John Philoponus, (6th cent. A.D.) and again with Robert Kilwardby (13th cent.) and Jean Buridan (14th cent.), the difficulties of this view were realized, and a new theory was proposed, which, in the form given it by the great Thomist, Dominic Soto (16th cent.), prepared the way for the Newtonian laws of motion. According to this new theory, the projectile continues to move not through any agency of the medium, but by a force (*vis*) given to it by the projector at the beginning of the motion when projector and projectile are in contact. This *vis* is an active quality which acts as the efficient cause of the motion, and which remains until destroyed by some resisting body encountered by the projectile.

Aquinas never accepted this impetus theory, although later Thomists, in their effort to answer the objections of Newtonian science, have adopted it.[21] For purposes of this discussion, however, I will concede that it is *not* inconsistent with Thomistic principles. Those who believe that it *is* would have to concede that in view of modern science and the Newtonian laws (a) either the theory of the action of the medium has to be saved in some new way, or (b) the entire Thomistic argument, as well as his theory of delayed hominization, collapses.[22]

Messenger and Dorlodot (on whom Donceel largely relies) revived the theory of delayed hominization, because it seemed to them to provide some Thomistic foundation for a theory of mediate creation of species by God through evolution. If, in human embryology, there is a transformation of an embryo living by vegetative life into a second embryo living with animal life and this finally into a truly human embryo by means of a certain power given to the vegetative embryo by the male parent, then what objection could even strict Thomist metaphysicians (who were in fact the most troublesome opponents of the theory of evolution, or of "the error of transformism" as they called it) raise against a theistic theory of evolution in which the Creator gave to lower species an instrumental power to transform themselves into ever higher and higher species?

As I have argued elsewhere, such theories of a special "evolutionary force" are not necessary for a satisfactory theory of evolution compatible with Thomist views on causality.[23] But, if we take such an approach to the embryological problem, how could we work out a theory? We would have to suppose that the vegetative embryo is living only a vegetative life,which of itself would never result in the substantial change necessary to produce an animal embryo living with sensitive life. It would, however, in addition to its vegetative soul, be endowed with an intrinsic instrumental power (*virtus*) given to it by the male parent which would bring about these changes. It would seem that this virtus would have to reside, at least principally, in the primary organ, first of the vegetative embryo, and next of the sensitive embryo. If it did not modify the activity of this primary organ, which is the prime mover of all the accidental changes within the organism, how could it guide these changes so as to prepare for the ultimate steps of substantial change?

Thus it would seem the two possible Thomistic theories would be:

1. Aquinas' own view that the male parent gives to the seminal spirit an instrumental power by which it is able (remaining a separate entity in contact with the maternal material) to act as the efficient cause to first form a vegetative embryo, then to transform this into a new animal embryo, and finally to perfect this embryo to the point that God, without a miracle, can directly effect the final transformation into a human person.
2. A modified Thomistic theory, by which the male parent gives to the semen an instrumental power by which it first forms the vegetative embryo, along with the embryo's own primary organ. This it also endows with the instrumental power which is, until that time, possessed by the semen (the semen then becoming ineffective and incorporated into the embryonic matter), so that this vegetative embryo, by means of its primary organ, is able to transform itself into a new animal embryo,whose primary organ, in turn, receives the instrumental power by which this embryo raises itself to the point that God, without a miracle, can directly effect the final transformation into a human person.

An Evaluation of this Theory in Light of Current Embryological Data

After having made clear exactly what this Thomistic theory implies, we are now ready to evaluate it in terms of modern embryological data so as to see how it must be modified if its fundamental philosophical principles are to be retained.[24]

1) The first obvious modification which is required respects the maternal matter. Aquinas supposed that this was the menstrual blood which was only inanimate, refined nutritional material. In fact, the mother's contribution is the *ovum*, which, as a part of her own body, is ensouled by her own spiritual soul. At ovulation it is separated from the mother's body and becomes a distinct, living entity, very highly organized, with its own primary organ (the nucleus). There is every evidence that this ovum is very close to readiness for rapid embryological development: (1) because it contains within itself a considerable amount of cytoplasmic matter sufficient to fuel it until implantation and development of the placental system, since only then will any other source of nutrition be available; and (2) because, in the nucleus, it has the power to produce the messenger RNA, by which it will guide the early stages of embryonic development up to implantation.[25]

In lower living things parthenogenesis is experimentally possible, and some believe that it occasionally takes place even in human reproduction, precisely because the ovum is haploid (has only one member of each paired set of chromosomes), but apparently this does not absolutely exclude development.[26]

Thus, while for Aquinas, the development *distance* which the efficient cause must overcome was very great, and which, therefore, required a considerable *time* before the maternal matter was ready for the human soul, modern biology sees this developmental distance as much shorter, because the maternal matter, the ovum, is already very highly organized, and therefore proximately prepared. Thus logically, we should expect that hominization should occur much sooner than Aristotle and Aquinas would have imagined. Of course this still requires an empirical determination of what exactly is the duration of this period.

2) A modification of the Thomistic theory is necessary, because we now know that the seminal fluid does not consist of a passive material (which is to be mingled with the maternal material) and active spirit, but material which is active by reason of the sperm, which, again, is already a living entity, originally part of the father's body, and living by his human life, which then becomes a separated entity living by its own very real, if brief and imperfect life. This sperm does not remain separate from the embryo as an agent transforming it, but fuses at conception with the ovum. This process of fertilization is not instantaneous, but is a fairly complicated one, which, however, ordinarily takes only a brief time.[27] Its result is twofold: (a) the sperm, which, like the ovum, is haploid, contributes the second set of chromosomes to the nucleus of the new, fertilized zygote, which thus has a complete set of paired chromosomes, half from the ovum, half from the sperm, thus constituting a new and unique set of genes, different from those in the cells of either parent; (b) the sperm by its entrance into the ovum, *initiates* the process of fusion of the two cells to form the new zygote, which at once begins to develop in the direction of a mature adult human being.

It seems plausible enough, therefore, that we retain the Thomist view that the semen (i.e., the sperm) is the *efficient cause* of the production of the new entity we call the zygote, and that it does this by virtue of an instrumental power received from the male parent. The empirical sign of its character as efficient cause is that the ovum remains in a resting state until the entry of the sperm initiates the fertilization process. That its power is instrumental seems consistent with the fact that the sperm is produced by the male parent as a functional instrument of self-reproduction, that it is an imperfect organism, haploid, and living only briefly, unable to nourish or reproduce itself. It also is evident that the sperm is able to perform its function in virtue of its own primary organ (its nucleus), which can thus be regarded as the seat of the instrumental power.

However, Aquinas' own unmodified theory is obviously disproved by the disappearance of seminal activity at the moment of conception. This means there is *no efficient cause for the rest of the embryological process.* Since "nothing can move itself," we thus have to resort to the second theory given above. By it the instrumental power resident in the nucleus of the sperm is transmitted to the nucleus of the zygote, which thus becomes the efficient cause of the embryological process. This nucleus, by its own inherent powers, is able to guide the vegetative life of the embryo only as regards vegetative functions, but, by its additional instrumental power, it will eventually be able to transform the vegetative embryo into an animal embryo, with some primary organ which (in addition to its own proper power of directing sensitive life) will receive the instrumental power to pave the way for the creative action of God.

3) Aquinas made no attempt to determine the primary organ of what he believed to be the vegetative embryo. According to Aristotelian botany, this was supposed to be located at the root end of a plant (analogous to the head-end of an animal).[28] According to modern data, it would clearly seem to be the nucleus of the zygote. But what is it, once that cell division begins? It is now known that when the ovum divides, all the nuclei of the daughter cells are essentially equal, and all the cells up to the blastula stage (when implantation or nidation occurs) retain totipotentiality (pluripotentiality). Consequently, during this period, identical twins may be produced if the mass of cells are divided, since each can develop into a complete organism; or separated cells may be rejoined and still form a normal organism. Hence, Diamond and others have argued that at this stage, no determinate individual exists, but rather, something like a colony of one-celled plants.[29]

The biological data, however, does not permit this conclusion.[30] From the moment of fertilization there already exists in the zygote (and this was probably already pre-determined in the ovum) a metabolic *polarity,* with the nucleus determining the upper pole of the metabolic gradient, and a *bilaterality* which will eventually be fundamental to the plan of the adult body. Consequently, as the first cell-divisions take place, there is already some differentiation in the cytoplasm of the daughter cells. They may be totipotential when separated, but as existing within the morula, they already constitute heterogenous parts. At this stage it appears that the maternal RNA produced in the cytoplasm by the DNA of the nucleus of the original ovum plays a regulative role, and the nuclei, with their new unique DNA, are still relatively quiescent. Nevertheless, it was the nucleus of the zygote which initiated the whole process, and it will be the new nuclear DNA which finally takes over the regulation of the development from the blastula stage on. Thus, during this intermediate phase, it is still the nuclear DNA which has ultimate regulatory control, although it permits the maternal RNA to play its own role. We ought, therefore, to hold that, during this time, the primary organ are the daughter nuclei, which originated from the nucleus of the zygote. Since all are essentially similar, they can be said to act collectively, although it is probable that some of them, or even one, located at the superior pole of the organism, has the dominant effect, and can be identified as the primary organ of the whole.

At the blastocyst stage, when implantation occurs, a patch of cells called "the primary organizer" appears on the posterior lip of the blastopore.[31] If this is removed, embryological development ceases, and if restored, it begins again. With its appearance, the totipotentiality of the cells ceases, and from that time on, differentiation of the parts of the organism is, for the most part, irreversible. Thus this "primary organizer" is clearly the primary organ of the blastocyst and is the epigenetic successor of the nucleus of the zygote, and of nuclei of the cells at the superior pole at the morula stage, as evidenced by the unbroken continuity of the polarity and bilaterality.

By the end of the second week following fertilization, the blastocyst has become the gastrula, in which the three basic body layers, ectoderm, mesoderm and endoderm, have differentiated. Out of the ectoderm, the nervous system, skin and other sense organs will form. (It should be recalled that for Aquinas, it is the sense of touch which is the basic sense determining animal life, and it is the character of this sense which is specifically human.) Before this week is completed, the *primitive streak* has appeared, which is the primordium of the central nervous system, and this already exhibits a polarity which indicates at which end the brain will be formed. From this period on, the development of the central nervous system with the brain as its superior pole progresses in a clearly continuous manner.[32]

Thus we can very reasonably interpret the biological data according to Thomistic terminology in the following manner: (a) The vegetative phase cannot last longer than two weeks in the human embryo; (b) Even in this stage, an epigenetic continuity can be traced between the nucleus of the zygote as primary organ to the primitive streak as primary organ of the animal phase.

4) Since the embryological data establish this epigenetic continuity between the primary organ of the vegetative and of the animal stage, this can be interpreted in one of two ways: (a) by the modified Thomistic theory, according to which these two organs are actually primary parts of two distinct substances, the first being transformed into the second by a substantial change, the efficient cause of which is an instrumental power with which the first primary organ was endowed by the sperm; (b) or by saying that the act of fertilization immediately produced not a vegetative embryo, but an animal embryo whose primary organ (the nucleus) is epigenetically and substantially identical with the primordial central nervous system manifested in the primitive streak.

The second interpretation seems far more plausible and economical. It is perfectly consistent with Thomistic principles, based on the following considerations: The sperm, as an instrument of the male parent who is genetically an animal, certainly has the power to produce a similar animal. Also, as was discussed above, the developmental distance to be spanned between the ovum and the zygote is very short, and consequently does not demand infinite power in the agent. In fact the first explanation may be eliminated as lacking any empirical confirmation and positing an unnecessary occult power in the first primary organ. It certainly lacks any authority from St. Thomas himself, since his explanation was quite different, and, granted what we know about the disappearance of the sperm, untenable.

5) Having eliminated on empirical grounds any reason to believe that the human embryo is ever ensouled with a vegetative soul, we now have to ask whether it has a merely animal soul during some period prior to hominization. The reason for such a hypothesis, as given by Donceel, would be that this period is necessary for the development of the cerebral cortex, i.e., for the elevation of the embryo from a low form of animal life to the supreme level of nervous organization required for the functioning of the internal senses of imagination, the *vis aestimativa,* etc.

Here it should again be recalled that St. Thomas himself believed that what is specific to the human sense organs is their high degree of neutrality, and that this is found primarily in the sense of touch. A man can be a man, can think and will, as long as he has the sense of touch, even if the other sense organs are lacking. Since, as we have already shown, Donceel cannot possibly be demanding the presence of the fully developed cortex for hominization, what is in question is the primordium of the specifically human capacity for the highest degree of sensitive life. Is there any reason to believe that this primordium is not initially present in the primitive streak of the blastocyst? We know that in the nucleus of the zygote there is already present all the *information* (order, or formal cause) and the inherent developmental power (efficient cause) to construct the human nervous system, including the marvelously complicated neuronic pathways of the cerebral cortex. This does not mean that the nucleus contains a preformed, miniaturized cerebral cortex. The nucleus is the primary organ of a total organism which develops epigenetically, each part of the system reacting on the others at every point of development and maturity. What it does mean is that an existential and dynamic continuity can be traced from the nucleus of the zygote to the cortex of the human infant. There is at all times a central organ maintaining life and producing development and differentiation, and this constitutes an epigenetic identity.

We must not merely understand the zygotic nucleus as a genetic "blueprint" and then argue, as some authors have done, that a "blueprint" is not identical with the building. The nucleus *does* contain a blueprint or exemplar of the adult in its genetic code. In addition, it has the active power to produce the finished building, and to produce it, not as something separate from itself, but as a transformation of the total organism of which the nucleus itself is a part. As we have seen, for a Thomist, this can mean only one of two things: (1) either the zygote is already informed by the substantial form or soul of the adult into which it will develop; or (2) the transformation results from an instrumental power with which the central organ of the zygote has been endowed. We have shown that this latter explanation is uneconomical and empirically unverifiable.

Consequently, we must conclude that no substantial change takes place in the animal zygote at hominization, so that it must have been hominized from the moment when fertilization was complete.

A Brief Consideration of Three Common Objections to Immediate Hominization

I will now deal very briefly with three objections which are commonly posed against immediate hominization:

1) Many authors,including Karl Rahner,are disturbed by the fact that a very large number of fertilized ova, perhaps as many as 50% or even higher, do not develop.[33] Does God create all these souls which are never able to live a human life? Others even argue that this logically leads to the absurd result that we should attempt to baptize countless minute zygotes or embryos, or that laws will have to be passed to protect them, or that few people believe that use of contraceptive devices, such as the pill or IUD, constitutes murder because they prevent implantation.

The answer to these objections can be found in a distinction of the concept "fertilized ovum." As indicated, fertilization is an elaborate process, which often proves unsuccessful. There is good evidence that, in most of those cases, where the "fertilized" ovum fails to develop into a viable fetus, this process has never been normally completed.[34] Since I am arguing that hominization takes place at the completion of fertilization, it need not be concluded that God creates souls for all these hapless abnormal "zygotes." It might be noted also that this type of argument would lead to a denial of humanity to those countless infants who have died in the past when infant mortality was often as high as 50%. The difficulties about the duty to baptize arise from antiquated views concerning the salvation of unbaptized infants that few Catholic theologians would now support. As regards abortifacient contraceptives, the issue has to be decided not on general public attitudes, often based on misinformation, but on an objective evaluation of the issue as to when hominization begins.

2) The argument against immediate hominization based on the phenomena of twinning and recombination of cells at the preimplantation stage has seemed very impressive to some theologians, including Paul Ramsey,and is supported by Diamond and Ransil with numerous subsidiary arguments (which I believe have been sufficiently disposed of in the foregoing interpretation of the continuity of development given above), which purport to show that the individual identity of the embryo is only established at implantation.[35,36]

The basic facts, as have been demonstrated, are that, even in the zygote prior to cleavage, some differentiation already exists, and this continues in the cell mass that makes up the morula. During this period, the cells have totipotentiality only in the sense that if one, or a group of cells are separated from the original organism they still retain the capability of developing into a second complete individual. Geneticists believe, on the basis of experiments with lower animals, that it is at least theoretically possible to "clone" new human beings from most of the body tissues of an adult human.[37] If this were to take place, when would hominization or ensoulment occur? Obviously, a Thomist must say that if at the moment there exists living cellular material sufficiently prepared for hominization, God, as the author of nature, will complete the natural process by the creation of a human soul. In such a case, the process is not that of true sexual generation (i.e.,the clone would not be the "son" of the person from whom the tissue comes), but constitutes a sexual reproduction like that found in lower living things.[38]

Consequently, an adequate explanation of the facts, an explanation which is both economical and in line with the general theory I have elaborated, would be to say that the zygote is already a human being, whose central organ tends to retain its cells in a coherent and unified body as cleavage proceeds and gradually causes them to differentiate more and more perfectly. However, before this differentiation is complete, the cells retain a certain totipotentiality, and if separated by some accident from the original body, they become a new substance with its own form, by a process analogous to asexual reproduction, budding or cloning. Since these separated cells are still as prepared to live, as was the zygote, at the moment of fertilization, God supplies the twin with a human soul, just as He did the other twin. Both twins are truly children of the male parent, since it is the instrumental power of his sperm which has *initiated* the development of both, one directly, the other (as a result of an accidental occurrence) mediately, but by a mediation which is very simple and brief. On the other hand, the view that individual identity is established only at the end of this period, when twinning becomes impossible, has to answer to very significant biological difficulties. (1) If, during this period, the morula or blastula is merely a mass of cells, lacking individuality as a distinct organism, what causes it to develop and differentiate according to definite laws, as we observe it does? (2) If, only after the twinning stage is passed, the single embryo, or the twin embryos now each become self-identical organisms, what produces this new individual unity in each? *Ex hypothesi,* this does not derive from an internal principle, since if it did, we would have to assume that one (or two) souls were already present *before* this stage. Clearly, also, it does not come from the mother, since there is no evidence that the mother is the agent of implantation. All the evidence indicates that the embryo implants itself. We are left with the possibility that it is God who individuates the cell mass by infusing the soul, but this is a recourse to divine intervention without attributing to biological processes their proper role. We can only conclude that the embryo at this stage already has its own individual vital unity, as all biological evidence indicates; but that in some cases, by accident, an asexual, "cloning" event occurs which gives rise to a second, new individual organism.

It seems to me that this difficulty about twinning arises largely from a rather mechanistic idea of God's action in creating the soul. Rather we must suppose theologically that, God, who controls not only natural but chance events, wills to create each human person, even when that person's body is produced by an embryological accident such as twinning, and hence, it is inconsequential just how the properly prepared matter for hominization results.

A similar explanation can be given to recombination experiments.[39] The individuality of the embryo depends on its primary organ. If cells are separated from the morula and then rejoined to it, they become a part of the living substance when they fall under the directive influence of the primary organ, as does a transplant into an adult body.

3) Some authors (notably Ransil) deny the individuality of the embryo because it is "symbiotic" with the mother.[40] They categorize it as analogical to a "parasite" or even a "tumor." To deal with such questions it is obviously necessary to distinguish between (a) parts of a single organism which are unified by a single "substantial form" manifested in a primary organ, and (b) distinct organisms interacting with each other, or a single organism reacting with its environment.

The biological data clearly indicate that no matter how intimate the reaction between the embryo (or fetus) and its mother, or maternal environment, the embryo is still a distinct organism with the capacity to develop into another member of the same species as the mother. The fact that the embryo is a member of the same species as the mother, makes it fundamentally different from a tumor or a parasite.

It is strange that Ransil and others continue to argue that the unborn embryo or fetus is not an individual because it is not independently viable. Obviously "independent viability" is a purely relative concept, not an absolute one, as is the notion of "human individual" or "person." No living thing has complete independent viability from other living things and the environment. The zygote, from the first moment after fertilization, has *some* independence in its life process, although it is minimal compared with the adult that it will become, but then even the adult does not have complete independence.

We can only conclude that according to present biological knowledge, theories of delayed hominization lack any solid empirical evidence.[41] Therefore, moral theologians should not use such theories as grounds for solving conflict situations in which the life of the conceptus and the mother are involved.

Footnotes

1. Aristotle's views are to be found in his *History of Animals, Parts of Animals,* and *Generation of Animals.* It has seemed to me unnecessary to document them here in detail. As for Aquinas the chief texts relating directly to this question (in probable chronological sequence according to James A. Weisheipl, O.P., *Friar Thomas D'Aquino,* Doubleday, Garden City, N.Y., 1974, 395 ff.) are as follows, with the most important in italics:
   (a) *Scriptum super libros Sententiarum* (1252-56): 2 dist. 8, q.1 a.4 ad 2 (demons could generate only by using human seed); dist. 18, q.1 a.2 (notion of *rationes seminales; dist. 18, q.2 a. 1 and 3* (mediate animation); dist. 20, q.1 a. 1 ad 3 (human

persons are uniquely intended by God); a.2 c. (reasons for sexual difference), ad 4,5,6 (semen is well-digested food); q.2, a.1 ad 1 and 2 (female is not unnatural; a. 2 c and ad 5 (imaginative power is in forebrain); dist. 30, q.2 a.3 (human souls share inequality of human bodies); 3 dist. 3, q.2 a.1 (male parent is agent of organization, female in preparing matter and nutrition); q.5 a.1 and 2 (Christ was animated at conception); 4 d.44, q.1 a.2 sol. 3 and a.5 ad 5 (embryo before animation will not be resurrected).

(b) *Summa contra gentiles* (completed 1264): II, c.58 (only intellective soul in man; c.68-69 (how soul is form of body); c.72 (soul is whole in the whole, and whole in every part); *c.86-89* (mediate animation); IV c.48-49 (Christ was animated at conception); c.81 (sex difference remains in resurrected body).

(c) Compendium Theologiae (possibly contemporary with *Summa contra gentiles*): c.92-95 (mediate animation).

(d) *Summa Theologiae,* Part III (1272-73): q.6 a.4 (matter of Christ's body existed before Christ); q. 27-28 (the Virginal Conception); q. 31 a.4-8 (conception of Christ); q.33 (Christ was animated at conception).

(e) *De Potentia* (1265): *q.3 a.9-12* (mediate animation); q.5 a.9 (role of cosmic forces in generation).

(f) *De Malo* (1266-67): q.4 a.3, 6, 7 (original sin transmitted seminally).

(g) *De spiritualibus creaturis* (1267-8): *a.3 ad 13* (life in embryo); a.4 and 5 (how whole soul is in the parts).

(h) *De anima* (1269); a. 8-12, especially *a.11 ad 2* (mediate animation).

(i) *Summa Theologiae,* Part I (1266-68): q.76 (union of soul and body); q.78 (powers of the soul); q.90-92 (creation of man; q.99 (Adam's children); *q.118, a.1-3* (mediate animation; q.119 (propagation of human body).

2. John Dedek, *Contemporary Medical Ethics,* Sheed and Ward, N.Y., 1975, c.7 "Abortion", pp. 109-135. Dedek takes the postion that "Contemporary theologians are only returning to an earlier theological position, saying that the prohibition of abortion is not an absolute one. Ordinarily the purposeful destruction of a fetus is morally wrong. But exceptions to this rule have to be made when a proportionate value, another life or its moral equivalent, is at stake" (p. 131), and quotes Karl Rahner S.J., Robert Springer, S.J., Richard McCormick S.J., and Bernard Haring, C.S.S.R. in support.

3. "Causality and Evolution" *New Scholasticism,* 39 (1965) 295-315; "Abortion: Mediate and Immediate Animation"; *Continuum 5* (1967) 167-71; "Immediate Animation and Delayed Hominization", *Theological Studies,* 31 (1970) 76-105; "Why is Abortion Wrong?", *America,* Aug. 16 (1975) 65-67.

4. A. Plé, O.P., "Alert au Traducianisme", *La Vie Spirituelle (Supplement)* 24 (96-99), (1971), 59-71. Plé does not say that mediate animation is more probable, but only that many current writers against abortion seem to use crypto-traducian arguments, forgetting the special creation of the human soul is *de fide,* but that there is no revelation concerning the moment of hominization. Plé continues the defense of St. Thomas' position maintained by several Dominican writers during the neo-Thomistic period, see e.g. H. M. Hering, O.P., "De tempore animationis foetus humani", *Angelicum,* 28 (1951) 18-19 who cites many other twentieth century authors of the same opinion, and M. Hudeczek, "De tempore animationis foetus humani secundum embryologian hodiernam", *Angelicum* 29 (1952) 162-181 who makes a strong argument on the basis of twinning. James J. Diamond, "Abortion, Animation and Biological Hominization," *Theological Studies,* 36 (1975), 305-324. Bernard J. Ransil M.D., *Abortion,* Paulist Press Deus Books, Paramus, N.J., 1969.

5. "Immediate Animation and Delayed Hominization", cited above n. 3, p. 101.

6. According to W. J. Hamilton, J. D. Boyd, and H. W. Mossman, *Human Embryology,* Heffer, Cambridge, 1957, "The primordium of the hippocampus is the first part of the human cortex to differentiate. It arises in embryos of about 12 mm" (p. 297). Such an embryo would be about 40 days old.

7. For Aquinas, as for most partristic and medieval theologians, this question was discussed in the context of the problem of the transmission of original sin, in opposition to Tertullian's *traducianism* i.e. the theory that the parents produced the spiritual soul of the child as well as its biological organism. For the history of this see A. Chollet, "Animation", and J. Bainvel, "Ame" in *Dictionnaire de theologie,* t.I, cols, 1305-20 and 967-1006 respectively. Also John T. Noonan Jr., "The Catholic Church and Abortion", *Dublin Review,* 261 (Winter 1967-68) 300-345.

8. Aristotle's theory is developed in *De Generatione Animalium,* II, 1, 733b, 24 sq. Aquinas did not comment on this work, but he constantly refers to it. What Aristotle meant by "epigenesis" (the term today is sometimes used rather vaguely, simply as the opposite of "preformation") was that the organism when first constituted as an individual need have only *two* differentiated parts, one of which then acts as the agent to differentiate the other parts out of the matter of the other which at first is only *potentially* differentiated.
9. *Scriptum super libros Sententiarum,* 3 dist. 3, q. a.1 and 2; *Summa contra gentiles* IV, c.48-45; *Summa Theologiae* III, q. 33 a.1.
10. *Scriptum super libros Sententiarum,* d.3, q.5 a.2 ad 3m: "An individual has its minimum quality in the first instant of its formation and animation, which is so small that it hardly exceeds the size of an ant, for Aristotle says in IX *De anim.* (*Historia Animalium* VII, 3, 583b 17-18) that when a certain woman suffered an abortion on the fortieth day of pregnancy, the body of the fetus was found to have all its members differentiated, although it was only the size of a large ant". Actually it would be about 13 mm. in length, i.e. 1/2 inch.
11. *Generation of Animals* I, 2, 716a 2 sq.: *Summa Theologiae* q.92 a.1 c. and many other places in Aquinas' works. On the role of the female parent in ancient embryology as *actively* furnishing the matter of the fetus and fostering its growth and development see Cletus Wessels, O.P., *The Mother of God: Her Physical Maternity,* Aquinas Library, River Forest, Ill., 1964, especially Section Two, Chapter III, 124-151.
12. "But nature never fails in necessary things: therefore the intellectual soul has to be endowed not only with the power of understanding, but also with the power of feeling. Now the action of the senses is not performed without a corporeal instrument. Therefore it behooved the intellectual soul to be united to a body fitted to be a convenient organ of sense. Now all the other senses are based on the sense of touch. But the organ of touch required to be a medium between contraries, such as hot and cold, wet and dry, and the like, of which the sense of touch has the perception; thus it is in potentiality with regard to contraries, and is able to perceive them. Therefore the more the organ of touch is reduced to an equable complexion, the more sensitive will be the touch. But the intellectual soul has the power of sense in all its completeness . . . Therefore the body to which the intellectual soul is united should be a mixed body, above others reduced to the most equable complexion. For this reason among animals, man has the best sense of touch. And among men those who have the best sense of touch have the best intelligence." *Summa Theologiae* I, q. 76 a.5 c.
13. See Elmar Klinger, articlo "Soul", *Sacramentum Mundi* (ed by K. Rahner et al) Herder and Herder, N.Y., 1970, vol. 6, 138-141.
14. *De Malo,* q.4 a.3,6,7,; *Summa Theologiae* III q. 31-35.
15. *De Malo, ibid;* Summa Theologiae I, q. 118-119.
16. "The likeness of the begetter to the begotten is on account not of the matter, but of the form of the agent that generates its like. Wherefore in order for a man to be like his grandfather, there is no need that the corporeal seminal matter should have been in the grandfather; but that there be in the semen a virtue derived from the soul of the grandfather throught the father." *Summa Theologiae,* I, q.119 a.2 ad 4m. However, Aquinas seems to admit that some part of the male seed mixes with the female, since he says (see following note) that the semen consists in two parts, only one of which is active. Consequently, the passive part must mix with the passive female seed.
17. Aristotle's theory of the semen and the vital *pneuma* which it contains is thoroughly discussed by A. L. Peck in Appendix B of his edition of *Generation of Animals,* Loeb Library, Harvard, 1953, 576-593 and is correctly reported by St. Thomas, *Summa Theologiae* I, q.118 a.1 ad 4, De Potentia q.3, a.9 ad 16 and elsewhere in the texts given above. It is also commented on by John of St. Thomas, *Cursus Philosophicus Thomisticus* (ed. Reiser, Marietti, Torino, 1933) II, iii q. viii, a.iii, 730 sq.
18. On the role of the menstrual blood see references in n.11 above. On the role of the male semen: "The power (*virtus*) which is in the father's semen is an intrinsic and permanent power, not applied from without as is the moving power in a projectile. Therefore the power in the semen remains effective, even when the father is removed to a distance. . . .Nevertheless, there is some similarity, since just as the finite power of the thrower moves the projectile only to a determinate distance of place by local motion; so the power of the parent moves [the fetus] only to a determinate form by

the motion of generation", *De Anima* a.11 ad 2.

19. "In perfect animals, generated by coition, the active force is in the semen of the male, as the Philosopher says (*Generation of Animals* II, 3); but the foetal matter is provided by the female. In this matter the vegetative soul exists from the very beginning, not as to the second act, but as to the first act, as the sensitive soul is in one who sleeps. But as soon as it begins to attract nourishment, then it already operates in act. This matter therefore is transmuted by the power which is in the semen of the male, until it is actually informed by the sensitive soul; not as though the force itself which was in the semen becomes the sensitive soul; for thus, indeed, the generator and generated would be identical; moreover, this would be more like nourishment and growth than generation, as the Philosopher says. And after the sensitive soul, by the power of the active principle in the semen, has been produced in one of the principal parts of the thing generated, then it is that the sensitive soul of the offspring begins to work towards the perfection of its own body, by nourishment and growth. As to the active power which was in the semen, it ceases to exist, when the semen is dissolved and the spirit thereof vanishes. Nor is there anything unreasonable in this, because this force is not the principal but the instrumental agent; and the movement of an instrument ceases when once the effect has been produced." (*Summa Theologiae* I, q. 118 a.1. ad 4.) There is a difficulty of interpretation in this text because Aquinas here seems to say that the menstrual blood is alive vegetatively before the action of the male semen, which is contrary to his statement in q.119 a.2, where he shows that it is nutritive material that has never yet been assimilated to the actually animated state. Peck (see note 17) above interprets Aristotle as saying it is alive with vegetative life, so that the male only raises it to sensitive life. John of St. Thomas (see reference in note 17 above) says also that it has an imperfect life. However, I believe that although Aquinas is not very clear on the point, it is more consistent to say that this nutritive material has never been actually alive, and that Aquinas when he says "the vegetative soul exists from the very beginning" means by "the very beginning" (*a principio*) from the very beginning of the action of the male semen, as he says in another passage:

   "Thus therefore through the formative virtue which is in the semen, after expelling the form of the [female] seed, another form is induced; and when this has been expelled, another is induced. And thus *first the vegetative soul is induced;* and then when this has been expelled, a soul which is both vegetative and sensible; and when this has been expelled there is induced not through the seminal power but by the Creator, a soul which is at the same time rational, sensitive, and vegetable." (*De Potentia,* q.3 a.9 ad 8.)

20. A. Rozwadowski A.J., "De motus localis causa proxima secundum principia S. Thomae", *Divus Thomas* (Piacenza), 42 (1939) pp. 104-113, attempted to show that the theory of *impetus* is to be found in St. Thomas, depending largely on the text from *De Anima* quoted in note 18 above. He was refuted by a writer (evidently M. D. Chenu) in *Bulletin Thomiste* 6 (1940-42) n. 351, and M. D. Chenu, O.P., "Aus origines de la science moderne", *Revue de Sciences Philosophiques et Theologiques,* 29 (1940) p. 206-217.

21. For example see Antonio Moreno, "The Law of Inertia and the Principle *Quidquid movetur ab alio movetur", The Thomist* 38, April 1974, 206-331. Moreno goes beyond the classical impetus theory, however, by showing that in Einsteinian physics all motion involves a relation between the moving body and the *field* in which it moves, which may be the solution to the Thomistic difficulty.

22. Messenger, E. C. "The Embryology of St. Thomas Aquinas", 243-258, and Canon de Dorlodot, "A Vindication of the Mediate Animation Theory", 259-283 in Messenger, E. C., ed. *Theology and Evolution,* Newman, Westminister, Maryland, 1949. Donceel in his article "Causality and Evolution" (note 3 above) seems to have first become interested in this whole problem by his effort to defend Teilhard de Chardin's evolutionary world-view in terms of Rahner's hominization theories.

23. See my article "Causality and Evolution", *The Thomist* 36 (April, 1972) 199-230, in which I argue that theories like those of Karl Rhaner, which posit a tendency of all creatures to transcend themselves, or of Teilhard de Chardin's universal "law of evolution" are uneconomical in explaining the compatibility of scientific theories of evolution and the principle of causality.

24. Besides the article of Diamond and the book of Ransil (note 4 above) and the book W. J. Hamilton, J. D. Boyd and H. W. Mossman (note 6 above) I have used Fracis G. Gilchrist, "A Survey of Embryology", Prentice-Hall, N.Y., 1968 for the current views

of embryologists.

25. Gilchrist, *op. cit.* p. 30-33, 43-44, 69-72.
26. *Ibid.* 65-66, 68-69.
27. *Ibid.* 60-69.
28. *De Partibus Animalium* II, c. 10, 655b seq.
29. *Gilchrist,* p. 5-17, Diamond, *op. cit.,* p. 311 f.
30. Gilchrist, *op. cit.* 62-65
31. Diamond, *op. cit.,* 314, n. 18
32. *Gilchrist, op. cit.* 260 ff. and Hamilton-Boyd-Mossman, *op. cit.* p. 47 and Chapter XII, p. 263 ff.
33. "For a few centuries Catholic moral theology has been convinced that individual hominization occurs at the moment of the fusion of the gametes. Will the moral theologian still have today the courage to maintain this presupposition of many of his moral theological statements, when he is suddenly told that from the start, 50% of the fecundated female ova never reach nidification in the uterus? Will he be able to admit that 50% of the "human beings"—real human beings with an "immortal" soul and an eternal destiny—do not, from the very start, get beyond the first stage of human existence?" Karl Rahner, *Schriften zur Theologie* 8 (Einsiedeln, 1967) 287, quoted by Donceel, "Immediate Animation" (reference in note 3 above) 99 ff.
34. See Diamond, *op. cit.* p. 311, note 12 says "Emil Witschi, "Congenital Malformations" *Proceedings of Third International Conference (Amsterdam)* (Excerpta Medica, 1970) . . . estimates that 58% of sperm-ovum conjugates never complete implantation; 16% terminate at conjunction, 15% never begin implantation, 27% are lost before the completion of implantation, and only 30% survive to birth. Many such failures would give a positive HCG test [a radioactive immune receptor assay test for pregnancy], despite the fact that differentiation and organismicization of somatic cells cannot occur due to defects intrinsic to the zygotes themselves. Hominizability, even *in potentia* does not exist." This, of course, argues that not every pregnancy is certainly a true human conception, but it does not agree, as Diamond seems to think that hominization is later than true conception i.e. a normal and perfect fertilization.
35. "The case of identical twins does, however, suggest a significant modification of any "proof" from genotype. If there is a moment in the development of nascent life subsequent to impregnation and prior to birth (or graduation from Princeton) at which it would be reasonable to believe that an individual human life *begins* to be inviolate, that moment is arguable at the appearance of a 'primitive streak' across the hollow cluster of developing cells that signals the separation of the same genotype into identical twins." Paul Ramsey, "The Morality of Abortion", in Daniel H. Labby ed., *Life or Death: Ethics and Options,* University of Washington Press, Seattle, 1968, 61-63.
36. "I simply cannot find in the biological order any reason not to distinguish radically and categorically between the preimplanted entity's vital capacity and that of the implanted entity. In short, the biologist holds that the numerous biological events converging in the general time area of the 14th to 22nd day weigh extremely heavily in any calculus of the beginning of the life of a homo". Diamond, *op.cit.* p. 316. Certainly he is correct in saying that the gastrulation and implantation stage is a very important moment in embryological development, as is birth, but this does not indicate that it is the *initiation* of the life of the individual. Ransil presents a still weaker case because he depends largely on the following argument: " . . . the product of conception and its mother exist as a single system in a symbiotic relationship, in which a host organism (the mother) harbors and nurtures a dependent organism (the product of conception). Contrary to what seems to be a self-evident fact, two equivalent individuals (in the sense of two independent beings of equivalent morphology and function) are not involved. Present is a coupled system of a mother and a product of conception" *op. cit.,* 82. But in this "coupled-system" are there not two *organisms?* Otherwise why call it "symbiosis"?
37. See James D. Watson, "Moving Toward the Clonal Man", *The Atlantic,* 227 (1971) 50-53.
38. For a Thomist there is a special difficulty in admitting that twinning involves asexual generation, since according to Aquinas original sin is transmitted by sexual generation. Would the twin then be "immaculately conceived"? But the same difficulty holds for the supposed possibility of a cloned human. However, contemporary theology understands original sin in a more inclusive way than did scholastic theologians, and would

interpret the phrase used by the Council of Trent when it said that original sin is transmitted *"per propagationem"* in a broad sense. Consequently it would seem that if a human being comes into existence by the action of sinful human beings, whether naturally, or accidentally (as in twinning), or artificially (as in cloning), this human would still share in the sinfulness of the human family. Christ would remain an exception because His conception is the result of miraculous Divine action, not of human power.

39. Diamond, *op. cit.,* 312.

40. "Perhaps the greatest difficulty for layman with the foregoing analogies and analysis will be his reluctance to view the fetus under the biological categories of parasite and tumor." Ransil, *op. cit.* p. 90 I would imagine most biologists, as well as laymen, might find this difficult! But then an analogy is between things which are "basically different, but in some respect the same."

41. Yet quite the contrary view has already been widely accepted by Catholic theologians who have not examined the evidence. For example William Allen, J.C.D. in "Abortion—Multiple Meaning", in *Pastoral Life,* Jan., 1976 45-51 writes: "At present, indications seem to be that medical science is moving away from the theory that the fetus is 'homo' from the moment of fertilization even though it is admitted that the fertilized human ovum is not the same as any other ovum or organism . . . Yet, the zygote does not take on hominization until the *primary organizer* appears on the posterior lip of the lower pole of the 'blastocyst'. Without this organizer there will be no further differentiation of cells into the essential organ systems proper to man" (p. 46). But what is it that differentiates the "primary organizer" itself?

Appendix II

Proposed Alternative Guidelines

In light of the observations about and objections (as presented in the text, Chapter V) to the Commission's recommendations, the following guidelines would be considered by the authors of this study as to be more in keeping with the Commission's own stated principles and in accord with the ethical implications of fetal experimentation analyzed in Chapters I-V.

1. Therapeutic research directed toward the fetus may be conducted or supported, and should be encouraged by the Secretary, DHEW, provided such research (a) conforms to appropriate medical standards; (b) has received the informed consent of the mother, the father not dissenting (when available and notified); and (c) has been approved by existing review procedures with adequate provision for the monitoring of the consent process.

2. Therapeutic research directed toward the pregnant woman may be conducted or supported, and should be encouraged by the Secretary DHEW, provided such research (a) has been evaluated for impact upon the fetus; (b) no additional risk to the well-being of the fetus will be imposed by research; (c) has been approved by existing review procedures with adequate provision for the monitoring of the consent process; and (d) the pregnant woman has given her informed consent.

3. Nontherapeutic research directed toward the pregnant woman may be conducted and supported by the Secretary, DHEW, provided such research (a) has been evaluated for possible impact upon the fetus; (b) no additional risk to the well-being of the fetus will be imposed by the

research; and (c) has been approved by existing procedures with adequate provision for the monitoring of the consent process.

4. Nontherapeutic research directed toward the fetus *in utero* may be conducted or supported by the Secretary, DHEW, provided (a) the purpose of such research is the development of important biomedical knowledge that cannot be obtained by alternative means; (b) investigation on pertinent animal models and nonpregnant humans has preceded such research; (c) minimal or no risk to the well-being of the fetus is imposed by the research; (d) the research has been approved by existing review procedures with adequate provision for the monitoring of the consent process; (e) the informed consent of the mother has been obtained; and (f) the father when notified has not objected to the research. No research should be permitted on a fetus-to-be-aborted that would not be permitted on one going to term.

5. Nontherapeutic research directed toward the nonviable fetus (living premature infant) may be conducted or supported by the Secretary, DHEW, provided (a) the purpose of such research is the development of important biomedical knowledge that cannot be obtained by alternative means; (b) investigation on pertinent animal models and nonpregnant humans has preceded such research and the research has been approved by existing review procedures with adequate provision for monitoring of the consent process; (d) the informed consent of the mother has been obtained, and the father when notified has not objected to the research; (e) the fetus is judged nonviable according to current scientific standards; and (f) there is no additional risk to the infant and no intrusion alters the duration of life. No research should be permitted upon a nonviable infant that results from an elective abortion which would not be permitted on a nonviable fetus resulting from a spontaneous abortion.

6. Nontherapeutic research directed toward the possibly viable infant may be conducted or supported by the Secretary, DHEW, provided (a) the purpose of such research is the development of important biomedical knowledge that cannot be obtained by alternative means; (b) investigation on pertinent animal models and nonpregnant humans has preceded such research; (c) no additional risk to the well-being of the infant will be imposed by the research; (d) the research has been approved by existing review procedures with adequate provision for the monitoring of the consent process; and (e) informed consent of either parent has been given, and neither parent has objected. No research should be permitted upon a possibly viable infant which results from an elective abortion which would not be performed on a possibly viable fetus which results from a spontaneous abortion.

7. Review procedures. Until the Commission makes its recommendations regarding review and consent procedures, the review procedures mentioned above are to be those presently required by the DHEW. In addition, provision for monitoring the consent process shall be required in order to insure adequacy of the consent process and to prevent unfair

discrimination in the selection of research subjects. In order to foster public understanding and make public attitudes known, appropriate provision should be made for public attendance at, and participation in the review process.

8. Research on the dead fetus and fetal tissue. The Commission recommends that the use of the dead fetus, fetal tissue, and fetal material for research purposes be permitted consistent with local law, the Uniform Anatomical Gift Act, and commonly held convictions about respect for the dead. Fetuses which result from elective abortion procedures should not be subject to research which is not permitted on dead fetuses that result from a spontaneous abortion. For the release of dead fetuses for research purposes, the permission of the mother or father is required if the fetus resulted from a spontaneous abortion; the permission of the coroner or medical examiner is required if the fetus resulted from an elective abortion.

9. The design and conduct of a nontherapeutic research protocol should not determine the recommendations by a physician regarding the advisability, timing or method of abortion.

10. Decisions made by a personal physician concerning the health care of a pregnant woman or fetus should not be compromised for research purposes, and when a physician of record is involved in a prospective research protocol, independent medical judgment on these issues is required. In such cases, review panels should assure that procedures for such independent medical judgment are adequate, and all conflict of interest or appearance thereof between appropriate health care and research objectives should be avoided.

11. The Commission recommends that federal legislation be passed which provides that:

No institution or individual person shall be required to perform or assist in the performance of any part of a health service program or research activity funded in whole or in part by the Secretary, DHEW, if the performance or assistance in the performance of such part if such program or activity would be contrary to the religious beliefs or moral convictions of said institution or individual person.

12. No inducements, monetary or otherwise, should be offered to procure an abortion for research purposes. Moreover, no inducements, monetary or otherwise, may be offered to procure living or dead aborted fetuses for research purposes. The research design should include an account of the current process used in the procedure to obtain aborted fetuses.

13. Research which is supported by the Secretary, DHEW, to be conducted outside the United States should, at the minimum, comply in full with the standards and procedures recommended herein.